LEC

Here are the facts about lecithin, the 'miracle' product of the soya bean which has been acknowledged as a vital factor in the prevention and treatment of heart disease. Apart from controlling cholesterol and strengthening the heart, lecithin also improves the nervous system, protects the liver and kidneys from disease and is an invaluable aid to slimmers.

By the same author
GARLIC

LECITHIN
The Cholesterol Controller

by

PAUL SIMONS

THORSONS PUBLISHING GROUP

This edition revised, expanded and reset 1983

8   10   9   7

British Library Cataloguing in Publication Data

Simons, Paul
  Lecithin
  1. Lecithin
  I. Title
  613.2'6   TX553.L/

  ISBN 0-7225-0864-6

Printed in Great Britain by
Richard Clay Ltd, Bungay, Suffolk

CONTENTS

Note to reader

Before following the self-help advice given in this book readers are earnestly urged to give careful consideration to the nature of their particular health problem, and to consult a competent physician if in any doubt. This book should not be regarded as a substitute for professional medical treatment, and whilst every care is taken to ensure the accuracy of the content, the author and the publishers cannot accept legal responsibility for any problem arising out of the experimentation with the methods described.

INTRODUCTION

For most of us, eating is a most pleasurable necessity; our food not only keeps us alive and healthy, it brings satisfaction and enjoyment. Eating provides the body with energy and a vast array of nutrients, some in very tiny amounts, to help the body's organs and cells perform their particular functions. If we eat the right sort of food in a well-balanced combination, so that our body receives all the nutrients it needs, then we will be fit, vital, active and really alive, able to enjoy life to the full and better able to ward off infection and disease. The human body is, however, a very delicate mechanism. Too much of one type of food or too little of another and that mechanism starts to go wrong. Sometimes this can be spotted quickly, when, for instance, too little vitamin C is present in the diet and scurvy forms on the skin, but often it takes many years for a faulty diet to become apparent. Then it is frequently too late to do anything, as is the case when too much of the wrong sort of fat is consumed and a fatal heart attack is the consequence.

This book is about fat and more particularly about a very special sort of fat – lecithin (pronounced less-ee-thin). Lecithin is special because it is a most versatile nutrient, a food capable of altering and affecting other fats in the human body in a beneficial way. Lecithin is capable of many things: some are well proved and documented, others have still to be conclusively confirmed, but sufficient evidence certainly exists to justify the claim that lecithin is a 'fat fighter'.

Lecithin, the fat fighter, means good news for slimmers, for lecithin not only assists the body to burn up fat, it also keeps it mobile within the body, thus preventing its accumulation in unwanted places where it causes such unsightly bulges. The role of lecithin as a fat fighter in the battle of the bulge is described in Chapter 7 but, important though this is to slimmers, it is certainly not the most crucial function of lecithin in the body. Too much fat does not just lead to overweight, since too much of the wrong sort of of fat can severely affect the health of the whole body, especially the liver and heart.

Fats have a vital role to play as part of a balanced diet. They are critical in the functioning of many organs and take very different forms. One of these fats, cholesterol, is believed by many to be a killer. Research and population studies throughout the world indicate that cholesterol is one of the principal dietary causes of coronary heart disease, but cholesterol can be controlled with lecithin.

Today, in the United Kingdom, more than four hundred people died from coronary heart disease. It was the same yesterday and it will be the same tomorrow. A large proportion of them are men who have not reached the normal retirement age. Many of them will be young men of thirty or forty years. Coronary disease accounts for more than 25 per cent of all deaths in the U.K. and although the increase has levelled out it is still an alarming figure. For men in the age-group forty-five to fifty-four years the death rate from heart disease is over 50 per cent. Staggering statistics – but even more sensational when the evidence points to the fact that many of these deaths are avoidable!

In all the industrialized nations of the western world, coronary heart disease is the most common cause of death, yet this disease was comparatively rare fifty years ago. In many countries people do not suffer from heart attacks and this is particularly true of primitive races. It is a reasonable conjecture that this disease is man-made – a disease of civilization – and if it is made by man it is logical to suggest that it can be prevented by man. That it is, in fact, avoidable.

One of the main causative factors of heart disease is too much cholesterol in the blood. It is deposited on the artery walls leading to a narrowing and hardening of the arteries and eventually to atherosclerosis.

In nature, lecithin occurs together with cholesterol in many foods. Lecithin is a biological emulsifier which keeps fats (including cholesterol) in suspension, allowing them to pass through the artery walls and preventing the build-up of hard deposits which choke the arteries and restrict the flow of blood. In this way lecithin can help to correct one of the principal causes of heart disease.

A high blood cholesterol level can be caused by eating too much saturated fat, but it is also closely associated with some of the other causative factors in heart disease. A survey carried out by the Institute of Directors Medical Centre in London showed that 30 per cent of smokers had high blood cholesterol compared with only 19 per cent of non-smokers. Other investigations have shown that regular exercise reduced the level of cholesterol in the blood (and increased the lecithin) and that lack of exercise raised it. Blood cholesterol can also be raised by obesity and stress, and when high blood pressure is accompanied by high cholesterol then the risk of death from heart disease is even higher.

Lecithin not only protects the heart and helps keep the figure trim, it is important for a beautiful skin. Many skin disorders such as psoriasis, eczema and some forms of acne are caused by faulty fat absorption and the skin relies on fat being fed to it by the blood, to remain clear, fresh and wrinkle-free.

Every cell in the human body contains lecithin and many organs need adequate supplies if they are to function properly. The liver, an enormously important organ, needs large quantities. Without lecithin in the bile, gallstones are formed. The heart and nerves both contain large amounts of lecithin and if they are to function properly this supply must be maintained.

The brain also needs a constituent of lecithin to enable it to function properly. During the last five years a considerable amount of research has indicated that lecithin can provide this substance, choline, in a form in which the brain can use it directly and it is believed that the memory can be improved and certain diseases concerned with old age can benefit from the inclusion of lecithin in the diet. These are significant new developments and research is still continuing to prove the initial findings.

Lecithin really is a most versatile nutrient, essential to every individual, vital for life itself. But what is it? Where does it come from? How does it work? How can it protect the heart, keep the body slim, the skin beautiful, the

nerves healthy and help avoid gallstones? Not all the
answers are known but there is evidence to indicate that
lecithin has a very significant role to play in human
nutrition. This book presents the arguments and facts
that lead many of the world's leading nutritional authorities
to believe that lecithin – the fat fighter – has a tremendous
potential for protecting the life and health of every one of
us.

1.
WHAT IS LECITHIN?

We are all aware that, under normal conditions, oil and water do not mix, yet for countless centuries cooks have blended fats and oils with water in baking and chemists have combined them in order to produce their suspensions, emulsions and creams. To achieve the desired results they used simple, natural ingredients in their recipes. Readily available foods such as egg yolk, buttermilk and seed germ oils contained a 'secret' that somehow held the oil and water together.

In 1850, a Frenchman, Maurice Gobley, discovered the substance which enabled the mixing (or emulsifying) of oil and water to take place. The substance had always been available, nature had seen to that. What Gobley did was to find out exactly what it was that made this phenomenon occur, and because he isolated the emulsifying agent from egg yolk, he gave to it the Greek name for the yolk of an egg – *lekithos*.

We now know this natural, biological emulsifier as lecithin. It has many applications throughout industry where its properties are used in the production of a variety of products, from margarine and chocolate to paint and cosmetics. More recently lecithin has come to be valued for its medicinal and nutritional properties. It can still be made from egg yolk but the most widely used and finest source for nutritional purposes is the soya bean.

The development of the commercial production of lecithin from soya beans began nearly sixty years ago in a Hamburg oil mill. For the first time it was possible to replace the expensive egg yolk lecithin with the more economical plant lecithin and a new technology was born. In the second half of this century much more has been learned about the technical and nutritional values of lecithin. In this book we shall be looking in particular at the nutritional properties of this most versatile nutrient, especially its relationship to cholesterol in the control of arteriosclerosis and heart disease.

A Miracle of Complexity
Lecithin is a food which belongs to a fat-like group of substances called phospholipids. It is a complex mixture of fats and essential fatty acids, together with phosphorus and two important (but difficult to obtain) B group vitamins, choline and inositol.

Although lecithin itself is predominantly a fat, it is its action on other fats or lipids in the body, especially in the blood (which is essentially an aqueous, or water, substance) that makes it highly valued as a nutritional supplement.

Fat is one of the essential constituents of the diet necessary for life and health. The others are protein, carbohydrate, vitamins, minerals and water. Throughout the western world the average diet contains too high a proportion of fat, particularly hard or saturated fat. In at least seven major countries, medical authorities, led by the American Medical Association and the Commission for Heart Disease Resources, have advocated a reduction in the total fat consumption *and* an increase in the ratio of polyunsaturated to saturated fat as a preventive measure against coronary heart disease, which kills one in four of those who die in the United Kingdom each year. The 1976 report of the Royal College of Physicians endorses this view.

Lecithin plays an important role in the metabolism of fat in the body. We shall be looking in particular at the way in which it reacts with one of those fats, cholesterol, which is believed to be the principal dietary factor in heart disease.

In order to fully understand the nature of lecithin, its action and uses, it is necessary to use certain chemical sounding names and phrases (the most important ones are explained in the Glossary) but one fact needs to be understood from the outset – lecithin is very definitely a food and not a drug or chemical. It has a very varied, and sometimes complicated, chemical structure but this should not be allowed to distract from the simple fact that it is a natural food of enormous value. Lecithin has been reported as being helpful in preventing the onset of arteriosclerotic conditions, narrowing and hardening of the arteries caused by deposits of fats especially cholesterol. Many doctors, including Dr Lester Morrison, author of *The Low Fat Way to Health and Longer Life*, consider this natural food to be a heart saver.

Lecithin is the name given to a group of substances, present in both animal and vegetable cells which are obtained mainly from oil bearing seeds such as the soya bean and from egg yolk. It is a mixture of several components, each having different chemical and physical properties, which biochemists call phosphatides or phospholipids. This means that they are fat-like substances combined with the mineral phosphorus. The phospholipids in lecithin are linked with choline and inositol, and these are believed to be very important in the control of cholesterol and in enabling the body to burn up fat to convert to energy.

Lecithin is also rich in essential fatty acids, especially polyunsaturated fatty acids, which are, as we shall discover later, particularly significant. Although these essential fatty acids are so important to the chemistry of the body they cannot be manufactured just by the body itself and so, just as with vitamins, they must be present in the food eaten.

Lecithin then, like vitamin B, is not a single substance but a complex of different nutrients, each with its own particular role to play in the body's chemistry. It should be understood, however, that the effect of lecithin is not explained by its content of choline, inositol, essential fatty acids and accompanying phospholipids, but by the substance lecithin itself, through its function in the body as a carrier of other compounds, as a transporter of fat, as a supplier of energy and as an essential component in the structure of body cells and organs.

A Natural Wonder

Lecithin occurs throughout nature in both the plant and animal kingdoms. It is present in all the cells and organs of the human body and is essential to life and health, for none of these cells and organs can function without the presence of lecithin. Because it is involved in many of the metabolic or chemical processes that take place within the body, it is of particular importance to those organs which have vital bodily functions to perform. It is essential in the structure of nerve tissue and to the proper functioning of the glands, including the sex glands. Adelle Davis, the world famous American nutritional author writing about lecithin in her book *Let's Get Well* says, 'In a healthy person, it forms 30 per cent of the dry weight of the brain and 73 per cent of the total liver fat, both of which are greatly decreased in persons dying of heart disease.'

Regular exercise, and the consequent improvement in physical fitness and endurance, increases the lecithin content of the muscles and of course the heart muscle, which has the highest lecithin content of all muscles, is the most difficult one to fatigue. It is reported that an increase of up to twenty-five per cent in the amount of lecithin in the flight muscle of birds, has been observed after regular exercise.

The lecithin content of tissue appears to remain remarkably constant even in cases of starvation, when ordinary fat and protein fall drastically. It is only when the body is extremely emaciated that there is a significant fall in the lecithin content of the cells.

Providing the diet contains the right components, the human body can produce lecithin. It is manufactured in the liver, passes into the intestine and is absorbed into the blood. Lecithin is essential to a great many of the body functions and in the structure of all body cells, so the body's demand for the raw materials needed to produce it is enormous. A deficiency of any one of them limits this production. It is fortunate that lecithin occurs in so many of the unrefined foods that we eat but unfortunate that many refined foods, e.g. white flour and hydrogenated (or hardened) fats, have had their store of of valuable lecithin destroyed by processing.

When, because of stress, physical or mental exertion, ageing or a diet containing insufficient of the component parts required by the liver to produce lecithin, there is a danger that a shortage of lecithin present in the body can seriously affect health and can be responsible for a build-up of cholesterol in the artery walls leading to arterio-sclerosis, one cause of ischaemic heart disease. In these circumstances a supplementary source of lecithin is required to keep the body fit and active.

There are many good food sources of lecithin. Unrefined or cold pressed vegetable oils and egg yolk have already been mentioned and others are nuts, whole wheat cereals, especially wheat germ itself, liver and beef hearts. However, a lot of our food only reaches us after it has been subjected to some degree of processing which is often responsible for the reduction or elimination of much of the available lecithin. For instance, vegetable oils are often treated with an alkali in the refining process, or the germ is separated from the grain in the milling process when flour is made. Sometimes the lecithin is destroyed or nullified in the kitchen, for example when an egg is fried in a saturated fat (lard). The one sure way to be certain that sufficient lecithin is available in the diet is to take a lecithin supplement and there are several on sale at all health food stores.

Lecithin Supplements

Nutritional supplements are intended to increase the available supply of active bodybuilding substances. They satisfy a particular nutritive requirement which may be lacking due to illness, deficiency disease, inadequate diet, and so on. They meet the increased demands of the body in time of stress, convalescence or after mental or physical exertion. Lecithin is a particularly valuable one.

The first lecithin produced by Maurice Gobley was made from egg yolk, as I have mentioned, and this is still a useful commercial source but, from the nutritional point of view, it has certain disadvantages when compared with lecithin obtained from vegetable sources. Egg yolk contains more than 6 per cent lecithin but it also contains large amounts of cholesterol, and cholesterol deposited in the arteries can, of course, lead to fatal heart disease. The lecithin-cholesterol ratio in egg yolk is such that the release of cholesterol is favoured.

Egg lecithin (or ovo-lecithin) contains fatty acids which the body needs but they are mostly in a *saturated* form and are less effective in lowering the blood cholesterol level than the *polyunsaturated* essential fatty acids which are available in lecithin produced from soya bean oil. Experiments conducted by Adams and Morgan indicate that polyunsaturated lecithin from soya beans accelerates the resorption of cholesterol much more effectively than saturated lecithin from egg yolk and also prevents the development of cholesterol-induced heart conditions in experimental animals. As early as 1954 Bloom, and later Bloomstraud, demonstrated that a significant amount of lecithin taken orally is absorbed into the blood stream intact. The ideal dietary supplement then is a vegetable lecithin, and one favoured by leading nutritionalists throughout the world for the control of heart and other diseases is a pure granular form of lecithin produced from the soya bean.

The soya beans which are the raw material of lecithin supplements come mostly from North America and Brazil and have the following approximate composition:

Protein	42 per cent
Carbohydrate	26 per cent
Fat	19 per cent
Water	11 per cent
Phospholipids (lecithin)	2 per cent

The beans are cleaned, partly dehulled, then split and rolled to form thin flakes. The oils are extracted from these flakes and a mixture containing soya oil and lecithin remains. This raw oil is then heated and water added. Under these conditions the lecithin swells to a jelly-like emulsion and can be split off from the oil using high speed separators. The water is then driven off as steam. The raw or crude lecithin which remains has the following approximate composition:

Phospholipids (lecithin)	60-70 per cent
Soya oil	27-37 per cent
Moisture	1½-2 per cent
Others	½-2 per cent

At this stage the lecithin is in oil form and is the type of lecithin used in the manufacture of capsules or which is spray dried onto milk powder, or other carriers, to produce some of the nutritional supplements that are available.

The quality and efficiency of lecithin used for nutritional purposes is dependent on the potency and composition of the phospholipid complex. The most suitable have a phospholipid content of 98-99 per cent and, more importantly, contain a high proportion of phosphatidyl choline, which is very close in character to the type of lecithin found in the human heart muscle.

If the raw lecithin is dehydrated, the soya oil removed and then blended, it is possible to obtain a granular or powdered lecithin which is very pure, and which contains a good balance of phospholipids. The very finest products have a total phospholipid or lecithin content as high as 98 to 99 per cent, the remaining 1 or 2 per cent being soya oil and water, plus some natural vitamin E.

We have already seen that there is another extremely important factor which just be taken into account when considering the biological effectiveness of lecithin, especially in relation to heart disease – that is the essential fatty acid content. The fatty acids in egg lecithin are mostly in a saturated form, but in a pure vegetable lecithin granule, as described above, 80 per cent or more of these fatty acids can be unsaturated.

The following table lists the main nutritional data available for a pure form of lecithin granules and, as a comparison, for lecithin oil. It is meant only as a guide. All lecithins are different and before choosing a supplement it is advisable to check the labels or, if these do not bear sufficient information, to seek the advice of the health store manager or the manufacturer.

Contents per teaspoonful

	Granular lecithin (3.5 g)	Lecithin oil (5 ml)
Calories	30	6
Carbohydrate and protein	–	–
Saturated fatty acids	400 mg	450 mg
Polyunsaturated fatty acids	2 g	1.35 g
Choline	100 mg	40 mg
Inositol	100 mg	18 mg
Phosphorus	110 mg	17 mg
Vitamin E	4 i.u.	2 i.u.

It is interesting to note that some of the vitamin E which was present in the soya bean has been retained by the lecithin. Vitamin E is a well known anti-oxidant and protects the lecithin from rancidity. It is believed that an increased consumption of polyunsaturated fatty acids increases the body's needs for vitamin E. With a lecithin supplement this vitamin E is already available and in the proportion decreed by nature to provide the anti-oxidant protection.

The type of lecithin used in the work of most leading researchers, and described by Dr Lester Morrison as the most effective natural cholesterol-reducing agent he had tested, is a granular vegetable lecithin with a high choline phospholipid content, having a high proportion of its essential fatty acids in a polyunsaturated form. This is the lecithin discussed in this book. It is a natural food supplement, a key factor in the control of cholesterol and is influential in many functions performed by the body.

Lecithin supplements can be purchased from your health food store and the range of products available offers a wide choice. There are different grades of lecithin with varying degrees of purity and effectiveness. If possible use only pure lecithin without any additions such as fillers or flavours; the very best and most effective is undoubtedly pure granular lecithin from soya beans.

Taking Your Lecithin Supplement

The simplest way to take lecithin granules is direct from the spoon or sprinkled onto breakfast cereals. They can also be added to hot milk drinks, made of course with skimmed milk.

Vidal Sassoon, in his entertaining book *A Year of Health and Beauty,* recommends lecithin as an ingredient of his famous vitality drink. This is prepared by adding one tablespoon of lecithin, two tablespoons of protein powder, together with a little bran and wheat germ in a liquidizer. Add a banana, two cups of skim milk and an egg. Blend for thirty seconds. This produces a high protein drink, ideal to start off the day. Orange juice or other fruits can be used in place of the banana and the egg is optional. The drink will keep in the refrigerator.

Whichever way you prefer to take your lecithin supplement, remember to take it regularly for the best results. It could save your life!

2.

THE VERSATILE NUTRIENT

The use of lecithin as a nutritional supplement is of comparatively recent origin. When the commercial production of soya bean lecithin commenced in 1930 it was used as a cheaper and more effective ingredient in a wide range of manufacturing processes, principally in the food and confectionery industries. The emulsifying properties and other physical characteristics of lecithin enabled food technologists to produce new and improved products with better flavours, textures and keeping properties. A brief examination of some of these characteristics will not only show how versatile lecithin is, but will also help in understanding something of the way in which it operates within the human body, what its principal roles are in the structure of cells and organs, and particularly in the blood.

The chemical structure of a molecule of lecithin is such that it can bind itself to the molecules of liquids which will not dissolve together, so that, for instance, molecules of oil or fat can be dispersed in molecules of water. Lecithin exhibits what technologists call 'surface tension lowering properties', enabling emulsions to be formed. In food production this capacity is used in many ways, for example it enables 20 per cent of water to be blended with 80 per cent of mixed fats to produce margarine, which is in fact a water in oil emulsion. Lecithin not only stops the fat and water from separating, it prevents 'splattering' when margarine is used for frying food.

In the human body lecithin allows particles of fat (or lipids) to be carried in an aqueous fluid, the blood, dispersing them as tiny particles, keeping them in suspension and preventing their being deposited on the artery walls.

The same physical characteristics of lecithin are being used by the body and by the producer of margarine, but in each case with different objectives and, of course, very different results.

In the production of chocolate, caramel or fudge-like confectionery, lecithin is extensively used to improve the flowing properties. Chocolate is a mixture of cocoa-butter, sugar, milk and water. When lecithin is added to this mixture it exerts a liquifying action, keeping it flowing by reducing the friction or surface tension between the otherwise incompatible ingredients. It also prevents the cocoa-butter fat and water from separating and stops the recrystallization of sugar in confectionery. In the same way that lecithin helps keep chocolate fluid during manufacture, it can help to keep the fats in the body moving, enabling them to be burned up as energy and avoiding the accumulation of surplus fat in areas where it forms unsightly bulges on the hips, thighs, upper arms, etc.

Another property of lecithin is used in the production of 'instant' drinks and beverages containing cocoa. Some powders have very poor wetting properties, they will not absorb water and so cannot be dissolved or dispersed easily. If a spoonful of cocoa powder is sprinkled onto cold water it floats on the surface for some time. By contrast, if lecithin is added to the cocoa, the powder is wetted immediately and is instantly drawn down into the cold water. Instant drink products contain mixtures of sugar, cocoa, vitamins, minerals and other nutrients which similarly exhibit poor dissolving properties. The addition of lecithin to this type of beverage enables the nutrients to be mixed instantly and be easily absorbed.

There are many other uses for lecithin in the food industry. Added to flour it enables better fat dispersal in baking. In bread making it assists dough to rise and improves freshness, makes sponges more soft and supple and improves the flakiness of Danish pastry.

In agriculture lecithin is used in the production of milk feeds for calves and piglets to improve fat absorption, and it improves milk yields in cows. Chickens display better growth and improved vitamin A storage in the liver if lecithin is included in the feed. It has also been found that disturbance of the development of chicks due to vitamin E deficiency can be eliminated only when lecithin is given at the same time as vitamin E. As soon as lecithin is omitted, the improvement resulting from the addition of vitamin E to the diet ceases. This demonstrates the action of lecithin as a catalyst in the absorption of fat soluble vitamins. Lecithin improves the absorption of vitamins A and E in humans and increases the storage of both these very important vitamins within the body.

There are of course other, synthetic, materials which are available, to meet the technical requirements of the food manufacturer, just as there are synthetic drugs to reduce blood cholesterol levels and prevent fat absorption problems. However, lecithin is a food and not a synthetic material and must definitely be preferable, in both the production of food and in nutrition, to other synthetic substances of widely varied chemical composition.

The dietetic uses of lecithin are based principally on its action upon fats within the body and its role in the structure of body cells. The human body is a very complex machine which draws on hundreds of nutritional substances in the food we eat and the air we breathe. These substances are all interdependent and a deficiency of any one of them can result in the malfunction of one or more of the complex chemical processes which take place in the body cells and organs. The chemical reactions which convert the nutrients into a form in which the body can use them to provide energy and growth or cell replacement, is known as the body's metabolism. Lecithin is extremely important to many of these metabolic processes, especially in the liver which depends on the conversion of fat to a form that can be used easily and efficiently.

Having mentioned the general uses of lecithin, I will now describe some of its specific properties as a nutritional supplement. Its actions in improving particular conditions and deficiency states will be discussed in detail in later chapters, but it will be useful at this stage to explain its benefits briefly.

Attracting Opposites

Lecithin acts as an intermediary, or emulsifier, between the blood and the water insoluble fatty substances carried in the blood stream. One side of the lecithin molecule attracts fat, the other water, which means that fats such as cholesterol are dispersed in the blood in small particles which can pass easily through the artery wall, into the capillaries and thus to the body cells. When insufficient lecithin is present in the blood, cholesterol is deposited in the artery walls causing them to harden and become less flexible. This is the condition known as arteriosclerosis.

The emulsifying and solubilizing properties of lecithin increase the digestibility and absorption of fats within the body. To the person on a weight reducing diet this means two things, first that the fat is burned up more readily and efficiently to provide energy, and, second, that unsightly deposits of fat are prevented from building up in undesirable areas. It also means that the body is able to use and absorb the important oil soluble vitamins A, D and E.

Gallstones are composed mainly of cholesterol and are formed when the bile fails to digest fat properly. Lecithin forms part of the bile and it is its emulsifying properties which help to prevent the formation of gallstones. Improved fat digestion also reduces the problems associated with diarrhoea and sprue.

Transforming Fat
Lecithin contains choline and inositol, the B group vitamins which play such an important part in the metabolism of fat within the body. In the body an enzyme, liathinose, is produced and this sets free choline which has the ability to alter fat into another form and thus prevent its accumulation in the liver, giving rise to the condition known as 'fatty liver'.

Improved fat metabolism by the addition of lecithin to the diet also plays its part in preventing gallstone formation and removing cholesterol from the artery walls, in arteriosclerosis and hardening of the arteries and blood vessels caused by advancing age. Lecithin also helps correct problems caused by deficiencies of choline and other nutritional agents in the kidneys.

Essential Fatty Acids Are Essential!
The essential fatty acids have an enormous part to play in

a great many of the body's functions and lecithin is of particular importance because it is an extremely rich source of the polyunsaturated fatty acids. It is believed by many authorities that these essential fatty acids in the form of lecithin are up to fifty times more active and available than the same fatty acids found in other sources.

The relationship between coronary heart disease and the amount of polyunsaturated fatty acids on the diet is very well documented. It would appear that the platelets in the blood become sticky when one of the essential fatty acids, linoleic acid, is not present in sufficient quantities. The platelets stick together forming blood clots or thrombi and these form an obstruction to the flow of blood through the arteries, cutting off the supply of oxygen and causing a heart attack.

It is also believed that multiple sclerosis can be helped by the addition of this same fatty acid, linoleic acid, to the diet.

It will be apparent, if the essential fatty acids are fifty times more active when taken as lecithin, that whatever can be achieved by supplementing the diet can be done much better if lecithin is used as the principal source.

Professor Hawthorn, who is Professor of Biochemistry at Nottingham University, is currently carrying out a series of experiments to determine whether lecithin is a more effective source of polyunsaturated fatty acids than vegetable oils.

The present evidence certainly suggests that soya lecithin is beneficial as a dietary component and is superior to vegetable oils in its ability to reduce cholesterol levels.

Skin Care

Lecithin is an effective ingredient of many cosmetic preparations. It is used for its technical properties which enhance the product and provide a natural emulsifier for creams and lotions. It also feeds the skin with fatty acids.

Many skin problems, however, are caused by the malfunction of some internal process. Beauty certainly is not skin-deep! Faulty fat absorption or fat transport via the blood can give rise to many skin diseases and lecithin has been reported to have beneficial results when used to treat psoriasis, dry skin, eczema, seborrhoea and some forms of acne.

Special Foods and Nerve Foods

Lecithin is used in many special diets and in diabetic foods. Dietetic drinks, pastry and semi-fat margarines are enhanced by the addition of lecithin. For diabetics lecithin provides an important supplementary source of energy and can prevent many of the secondary symptoms which often accompany diabetics, such as fat accumulation in the liver and rises in the level of blood fat and cholesterol.

Restoring Energy

In Germany large quantities of lecithin are consumed and it is appreciated for its energy restoring properties. It has been shown in experiments that athletes recover more quickly after training when they take lecithin regularly. People who are subjected to stress, heavy physical labour or concentrated mental activity will also find lecithin very beneficial.

Many sportsmen and body builders take lecithin as a supplement to help keep the heart and circulation healthy and to metabolize fats. Active show business personalities are also known to take lecithin supplements. Tommy Steele says it helps to keep him fit and healthy and has used it on medical advice to reduce his blood cholesterol levels. Michael Crawford, star of 'Barnum', is reported to take lecithin to help keep his muscles in tone and there are many others, such as Cary Grant, who believe it helps to keep them fit and vital.

The nerves contain a lot of phospholipids similar to those in soya lecithin. If the levels fall too far, stress conditions, nerve strain, irritability, insomnia and nervous debility may follow. Excessive mental exertion can also lead to similar results if sufficient lecithin is not made available to protect the nerves.

Lecithin certainly deserves its reputation as a most versatile natural food supplement. Research is continuing throughout the world into the nutritional benefits of lecithin. Much more has still to be learned or confirmed, but it is already clear that the substance discovered by Maurice Gobley is more than just a technical aid to emulsifying oil and water. It can be a life-saver.

Brain and Memory
During the last five years scientists have discovered that lecithin in the diet can have a direct effect on the functioning of the brain. Experiments have indicated that memory can be improved in the short term and there are considerable hopes that continuing research will indicate that a whole new area of therapy is likely to develop using the natural properties of lecithin in the treatment of brain disorders.

3.

FACTS ABOUT FATS

It will already be obvious that when lecithin is referred to as 'the fat fighter' there is more than one type of fat which has to be considered. Fighting the fat that leads to excess weight problems is very important not just to preserve a trim figure and good looks but also to prevent the medical problems caused by obesity. Too much fat in the diet adds weight, but even more dangerous than the fat which can be seen are the unseen fats which tend to raise the cholesterol level in the blood. Of course, fat is not all bad – it is essential for the maintenance of good health in the human body. Lecithin is itself a fat, and a very important one because of the part it plays in the metabolism of other fats and the control of cholesterol.

The term 'fat' includes oils, which are really fats that are liquid at normal temperatures. Edible oils and fats, or to give them their more scientific name, lipids, are important to health and are an essential part of the diet. They are found in many animal and plant foods and are used by the body in various ways.

1. They contribute a very concentrated form of energy. One gram of fat provides nine energy giving calories, this compared with four calories per gram for protein and carbohydrates. The energy from fat is released more slowly than that from protein or carbohydrate, so this, together with the high calorie content, makes it useful in reducing the bulk of the diet, as less weight of food needs to be consumed for the same calorie intake. All fats, whether of animal or plant origin, contribute the same energy value but it is important to remember that they perform very differently within the body.

2. They provide the body with oil-soluble vitamins and other nutrients.

The important oil-soluble vitamins A, D, E and K are

present in the fats we consume and they also contain essential fatty acids. The body cannot manufacture these oil-soluble vitamins and fatty acids unless the basic materials are obtained from fat-containing food in the diet.

3. Fats improve the palatability of food. The taste and texture of food is improved by fats, which make it more interesting and enjoyable to eat. Because fat acts as a lubricant it makes food easier to swallow. Fat, of course, adds variety to the methods which can be used in cooking. Fat foods are more satisfying or filling than other foods. This is because fat is digested more slowly and the stomach takes longer to empty – consequently the energy is available over a longer period than with, for instance, carbohydrates which are burned up very quickly.

4. Most of the fat in the body is depot or storage fat. This fat is available to meet the body's energy demands, but it performs other valuable functions. It helps to conserve body heat and it acts as a padding for the vital organs, protecting them from shock and injury. Fat also serves as an intestinal lubricant to moisten waste matter and facilitate its elimination from the system.

Only about half of this depot fat is stored under the skin. The rest is distributed throughout the body, a lot of it surrounding and protecting the kidneys and intestines. Whilst some depot fat is normal and varies from one individual to another, obesity is often defined as the condition which exists when over 30 per cent of the body weight is fat.

5. Fat builds body cells and plays a vital role in many bodily functions. In terms of quantity the body has a lot of depot fat, but in terms of quality the fats which are most important are those responsible for helping to build the body cells and tissues. These are much more complex structural fats and lecithin is one of the most important of them.

Fat is essential to health but it is important that the body receives the right type of fat. All food fats are made

up from glycerol and fatty acids. The most common type
of fats are the triglycerides in which one unit of glycerol is
combined with three fatty acids. It is the nature of the
fatty acids which determines whether a fat is a saturated
fat or an unsaturated fat.

Two Types of Fat

In simple terms there are two kinds of fat, saturated fat
and unsaturated fat. Saturated fats are usually of animal
origin and are hard or solid at normal temperatures.
Good examples are butter, cheese, lard, hard margarine,
meat fat and eggs, especially the egg yolk. These are the
fats which tend to raise the blood cholesterol level. Foods
such as chocolate, ice cream and many commercially
produced cakes and pastries contain a lot of saturated fat.

Unsaturated fats fall into two categories, mono-
unsaturated and polyunsaturated. The mono-unsaturated
fats have little or no influence on blood cholesterol
levels. They are neutral, neither increasing nor decreasing
the levels. These fats are sometimes hard and sometimes
soft, or they may be a combination of both. They are
found in a variety of foods such as poultry, olive oil,
peanuts and almonds. They are important because they
enter into many vital bodily functions, even though they
have no effect on blood cholesterol.

The polyunsaturated fats are the ones that are really
important. They help reduce blood cholesterol levels,
enter into a wide range of functions performed by the
vital organs and are essential for the building of new body
cells. These fats are soft fats, usually oils of vegetable or
fish origin. Examples are soya oil, corn oil, sunflower and
safflower oil and seeds, fish and fish liver oils. There are
now several special brands of margarine and salad dressing
which contain polyunsaturated fats and these can be
purchased at most supermarkets and all health food stores.

One of the richest and best sources of polyunsaturates
is lecithin, for lecithin contains them in the form of
phospholipids, which means that they are readily available
to be used in a wide spectrum of activities concerned with
the metabolism of fat, especially cholesterol. Professor
H. M. Sinclair, the Director of the International Institute

of Human Nutrition and for many years one of Britain's leading nutritional authorities, believes that the poly-unsaturated fatty acids in the form of pure lecithin can be up to fifty times more active in correcting fatty acid deficiencies than when taken as ordinary oils or fats.

The reason some fats are saturated and others poly-unsaturated is because of their chemical structure. All fatty acids (there are about forty of them) consist of the same three elements – carbon, hydrogen and oxygen linked together to form chains of molecules. In saturated fats the carbon part is joined to as many hydrogen atoms as it can hold so that there are no open links in the chain. This makes them hard at normal temperatures and incapable of reacting with other elements in the body in the way in which the polyunsaturates do.

The unsaturated fats have some open links left in the chain of elements because they do not hold as many hydrogen atoms as the saturated fats. This enables them to be joined up with other substances in the body and makes them capable of being absorbed. The unsaturated fatty acids which have the greater number of open-ended links in the chain are the polyunsaturates.

The essential polyunsaturated fatty acids are linoleic acid, linolenic acid and arachidionic acid. They are occasionally referred to as vitamin F but, although they are very similar in many respects to the vitamins, they are not vitamins in the true sense and the term vitamin F is not now used by nutritionists.

Most dietary fats consist of a combination of both saturated and unsaturated fats. The following table lists some common oils and fats in descending order of unsaturation (i.e. softness). Those at the top of the list contain a very high proportion of polyunsaturates, those nearer the bottom are very saturated (hard).

Safflower oil
Sunflower oil
Corn oil
Soya bean oil
Wheat germ oil
Lard

Hard margarine
Butter
Cocoa butter

Hard margarine is made from liquid oils which have been hardened by a process known as hydrogenation but it is possible to buy special margarines with large amounts of polyunsaturated fatty acids. This type of product is much better for health than other types and, if possible, should always be used instead of hard margarines and butter in cooking or for spreading.

The problem of hydrogenation of oils is important because once an oil, even a vegetable oil, has gone through this process it becomes saturated. Polyunsaturated oils tend to go rancid more quickly than saturated ones and this is especially so of oils which have had the naturally occurring vitamin E removed by processing. It is the well-known anti-oxidant properties of vitamin E that protects natural vegetable oils from rancidity, but the vitamin is easily destroyed by heat or chemical processing in the refining of oil. It is always preferable to obtain oils which have have been cold-pressed so that the vitamin E is preserved.

To prevent rancidity occurring and to extend the shelf life of manufactured products, many oils *are* hydrogenated. This involves introducing extra hydrogen into the fat, so that when it is absorbed some of the open links in the fatty acid chain are closed. This changes the polyunsaturated oil into saturated oil. It is not always possible to tell from reading the label whether a product contains oil which has been hydrogenated. Even margarines which claim to be made from vegetable oils can contain hydrogenated oils and so, instead of being rich in polyunsaturates as might be expected, they have become saturated and have the same adverse effect on blood cholesterol levels as animal fat products.

Generally speaking, the more polyunsaturated a fat is, the more easily it is oxidized. Unsaturated fatty acids increase the body's demand for anti-oxidants. In pure, granular, vegetable lecithin and in unhydrogenated vegetable oils there will be sufficient natural vitamin E present for most needs, but it is advisable to increase the supply of anti-oxidants when any attempt is made to replace saturated fats by polyunsaturated ones.

The Right Kind of Fat

Research and experience teach us that too much fat causes overweight and too much of the wrong sort of fat can lead to excess cholesterol and other fats being present in the blood. The answer, though, is not to eliminate fat from the diet. What is required is a balanced diet, one that will avoid the dangers of too much weight and protect the heart and other organs from excesses. To do this it is necessary to understand the facts about fats which have been presented in this chapter. The shopper or cook can see many fats such as butter, lard, margarine and knows that cooking oil is really a liquid fat. These fats are visible but, in addition, there are other invisible fats present in many foods. Most fruits and root vegetables, such as potatoes, contain very small amounts of fat, while at the other end of the scale cheese, chocolate and potato crisps are very oily foods with a high saturated fat content.

To protect the body from the dangers of excess fat it is not sufficient merely to add vegetable oils to the diet. It is equally important that they be used to replace animal fat and that the total consumption of fat is reduced. Hints on what to avoid and how to substitute dangerous fats with safe ones appear in another section, together with recipes for low saturated fat, cholesterol free diets. But listed below are some general guidelines to help plan a safe and healthy diet.

1. Reduce the amount of animal fat, cut excess fat from meat and eat less egg yolk.
2. Eat more poultry and fish.
3. Grill rather than fry and if you do fry use a vegetable oil.
4. Avoid the use of butter for spreading and baking; use a soft margarine rich in polyunsaturates.
5. Eat more fruit and vegetables of all kinds.
6. Take a regular daily supplement of pure lecithin, preferably in granular form.

4.
CONTROLLING CHOLESTEROL

The word 'cholesterol' has occurred repeatedly through-out this book and most of the comment has been pointing out the dangerous nature of the substance. It is without doubt the principal dietary cause of many diseases of the civilized nations of the world – the villain that afflicts us with heart disease, strokes and hardening of the arteries, that builds gall-stones and causes skin diseases. What is more, the dreaded substance seems to be present in so many of the foods that we enjoy: eggs, butter, cheese, meat, chocolate all add to the body's store of cholesterol. But is it all bad? Like so many other things, cholesterol only becomes a problem when it is present in our body in an unbalanced state. Unbalanced does not just mean too much cholesterol, it also means too little of the fat fighter – lecithin. For cholesterol is a fatty substance requiring lecithin to transfer it into the form required by the body for use in building cells and providing energy.

Countless experiments have contributed an enormous amount of evidence linking raised cholesterol levels in the blood with the development of various forms of arteriosclerosis. The report of the Royal College of Physicians into coronary heart disease, which has already been mentioned, adds further weight to the belief that there is a direct link between high blood fat levels, especially cholesterol, and heart disease. It is worth examining the nature of cholesterol and the way in which it acts for good and for bad within the human body.

The word cholesterol (like lecithin) is derived from Greek. *Chole* is the Greek word for bile and *sterol* the Greek for solid. Cholesterol, then, becomes a word meaning a solid, wax-like fat which is found in abundance in the bile. In fact, gallstones consist largely of cholesterol. Chemists describe cholesterol as a fatty alcohol which is white, tasteless and odourless and which will not dissolve in water. It is found in all animal fats and oils, in milk,

cheese, egg yolk, meat and some fish. The following table
gives the approximate cholesterol content of some
common foods.

milligrams per 100 grams (4 ounces)

Milk and milk products

Milk, whole	11
Milk, skimmed	3
Milk, condensed, evaporated	33
Single cream	66
Double cream	135
Cheese: Cheddar, Edam	100
Cream cheese	120
Cottage cheese	15
Cheese spread	65
Butter	250
Ice cream	45
Yogurt, low fat	8

Meat and fish (without bone)

Beef	70
Chicken, turkey	80
Lamb	70
Pork	70
Kidney	375
Liver	300
Crab	100
Oysters	50
Lobster	85
Wet fish	60

Sundry foods

Egg yolk	1500
Egg white	–
Vegetable oil	–
Special polyunsaturated margarines	–
Sponge cake	240
Fruit and vegetables	–

Even if the diet contains no cholesterol at all, it will still be
manufactured by the body. The liver is the organ which is

most concerned with the metabolism of fat in the body and it provides most of the cholesterol contained therein. But other organs and nearly all cells produce cholesterol so, even if all the dietary sources were eliminated, the body would still contain cholesterol which would find its way into the blood. The body uses fats to form cholesterol, but carbohydrate and even protein are also converted by the liver into cholesterol. Under normal conditions the body's mechanism produces more cholesterol than it receives directly from the diet and diets high in refined starches and sugar add considerable amounts of cholesterol to the blood. The body of a normal individual contains about 6 ounces (175g) of cholesterol.

If the diet is rich in foods containing polyunsaturated fatty acids then it will favour the production of cholesterol in a form that is more soluble and easier to emulsify within the blood; and, of course, if foods with a high cholesterol content are avoided, the body has a better chance of absorbing the cholesterol which it manufactures itself.

No substance in the body is completely independent of others and cholesterol is no exception to this rule. It cannot pass directly from the stomach or liver into the blood stream and body cells without other substances being available to alter its form in such a way that it can be absorbed. One substance more than any other is required by the body to convert cholesterol into a useable and helpful substance. That substance is lecithin. Cholesterol, just like any other fat, will not mix with water, and the blood is chiefly composed of water. Unless cholesterol is emulsified it will remain within the arteries, for the passages which carry blood from the arteries to the body cells (the capillaries) are very small and the relatively large lumps of cholesterol will not pass through them. Eventually the cholesterol becomes deposited on the walls of the arteries, and blocks them, giving rise to the condition known as arteriosclerosis. Lecithin is a natural, biological emulsifier and breaks down the particles of cholesterol into smaller units so that they can pass through the arteries and into the body cells.

The Benefits of Cholesterol

Cholesterol is a perfectly natural substance essential to the body. It only becomes dangerous when it is present in excess amounts and insufficient lecithin is available to convert it into energy and to use it in the structure of body cells. Before considering the harmful effects of cholesterol let us first consider its beneficial action within the human body.

As with other fats in the body, cholesterol is used to build cells. Body cells are constantly dying and need to be replaced. Cholesterol is present in the great majority of body cells. The adrenal, pituitary and sex hormones are all made with the help of cholesterol and it would appear that it cannot be replaced in the glands, once it has been used, without the presence of pantothenic acid. The endocrine glands use cholesterol to produce some of the steroid hormones.

The bile acids, which are essential for digesting and absorbing fats in the intestine, contain appreciable quantities of cholesterol and lecithin. When the cholesterol and lecithin are in balance fats are digested and absorbed without difficulty. If the cholesterol/lecithin balance is upset, then the cholesterol is precipitated out and forms into gallstones.

Vitamin D is sometimes referred to as the 'sunshine vitamin'. When the skin is exposed to sunlight the body has a mechanism which enables cholesterol to be converted into vitamin D. This vitamin is necessary for the absorption of calcium and phosphorus which play an important part in the formation of bones. So, indirectly, choleserol is necessary for strong bones.

Cholesterol appears to be particularly concentrated in the brain. Its function here is not fully understood but it would seem that in times of tension and stress the central nervous system calls on the body for extra supplies of cholesterol.

Another vital function of cholesterol is as a lubricant for the arteries. The heart pumps blood through the body at an incredibly fast speed. This very vigorous action would damage the walls of the blood vessels if it were not for the presence of liquid derivatives of cholesterol. To produce these derivatives the body combines cholesterol and lecithin and together they enter the blood stream and lubricate the arteries to prevent them from damage.

So cholesterol is not all bad. The cholesterol producing mechanism in the body was designed by nature because the substance is required in so many ways and it is only when too much cholesterol is present (especially if lecithin is low), that the problems arise.

The Dangers of Cholesterol

The heart, a fantastic organ about the size of a fist, pumps blood through the body at a terrific speed. During a normal lifetime about fifty million gallons of blood are pumped through the heart, carrying oxygen and nutrients to all parts of the body. Blood consists of water containing corpuscles and nutrients. Some of these nutrients are soluble, others are not. Among the insoluble substances transported by the blood to organs, cells and tissues, are the fats. Fats, as we know, are insoluble in water and need an emulsifier to hold them in suspension. The principal emulsifier is lecithin. Cholesterol is one of the fatty substances carried by the blood and if there is insufficient lecithin to form an emulsion in the blood, then it is deposited on the walls of the arteries. Eventually this build-up of cholesterol forms a hard core on the inside of the artery and is joined with other fats. The arteries become less elastic and flexible, they grow harder and narrower and impede the flow of blood. This is the condition known as arteriosclerosis. When it occurs in the coronary arteries, which carry the blood to the heart, the disease is known as atherosclerosis.

Arteriosclerosis can lead to many complications. By restricting the supply of blood to the eyes it can hasten the onset of cataracts; it can cause cramp, pain, coldness and discomfort in the legs, feet and hands; in the brain it can lead to forgetfulness and confusion and sometimes to strokes; in the heart it causes angina and eventually it can lead to death from coronary heart disease.

Studies of populations all over the world have shown a strong relationship between the level of cholesterol in the blood and the incidence of coronary heart disease.

Furthermore these studies have indicated that there is a direct link between the percentage of calories obtained from saturated fats in the diet and blood cholesterol levels. In Japan it is estimated that only 3 per cent of calories are from saturated fats and the rate of death from heart disease in men is thirty cases per thousand. In America 17 per cent of calories are from saturated fat and the rate of death is eighty per thousand men. In Finland where 22 per cent of calories are from saturated fat the rate is a hundred and twenty cases per thousand men.

Dr R. I. Jones of Chicago University, reporting on a series of studies relating to heart disease, lists the major causative factors in men in the following order.

1. Age
2. *Blood cholesterol*
3. Number of cigarettes smoked
4. Hypertension
5. Abnormal heart conditions
6. Body weight

He also reports that the severity of the arterial disease is related to the level of blood cholesterol.

In another well-known study, Professor J. N. Morris found that among London busmen those with the highest blood cholesterol levels had a coronary heart disease rate four times greater than the group with the lowest levels.

Tests carried out in Massachusetts covered five thousand men and women over a period of twenty years and showed that men under the age of forty-four years who had a high blood cholesterol level had a five times greater risk of coronary heart disease than those with a low cholesterol level. The risk factor for women was about the same, although the age of risk was fifty-five.

In early 1981 the *New England Journal of Medicine* reported the Western Electric Study. This was a long-term study involving 1,900 middle-aged men. The study, which was supported by the American Heart Association, looked into the effect of diet on serum cholesterol levels and deaths from coronary heart disease. It is a long-term study covering twenty years and is one of the most thorough investigations into the association between diet, cholesterol and heart disease ever to be carried out.

In its summary it reports that 'the results support the conclusion that lipid composition of the diet affects serum cholesterol concentration and the risk of coronary death in middle-aged American men.'

The blood cholesterol level is determined by weighing the total cholesterol in a given quantity of blood. A level over 250 milligrams per 100 millilitres of blood is considered high and it is often recommended that the level should be kept below 220 milligrams per 100 millilitres.

The amount of cholesterol present in the blood is an indicator that it is being deposited on the artery walls. Figures of deaths among men aged thirty to forty from coronary heart disease suggests that the deposits of cholesterol start to form at a relatively early age. Examination of the arteries of young men of twenty years who have been killed in road accidents, but who were otherwise healthy, has revealed that the porridge-like deposits of cholesterol and other fats are already significant and they continue to increase with ageing.

High blood cholesterol is only one factor producing heart disease. Other contributory factors are cigarette smoking, lack of exercise, obesity, stress and high blood pressure, and in all these instances cholesterol may be exerting an adverse influence. The survey of the Institute of Directors Medical Centre in London has shown that 30 per cent of smokers had cholesterol levels over 270 milli-grammes per 100 millilitres, against 19 per cent for non-smokers.

Experiments have shown that regular exercise can reduce blood cholesterol levels by up to 25 per cent and regular exercise is almost universally recommended as a preventative measure against the risk of heart disease. Overweight is a well known cause of heart disease. It is a condition which often leads to high blood pressure or diabetes. In diabetics there is often a high blood cholesterol level and high blood pressure can help to force cholesterol and other fats into the artery walls, causing arteriosclerosis.

Stress may also cause an increase in blood cholesterol

levels, as shown by tests carried out on students immediately before examinations, when the levels were raised compared to those in the same students some weeks earlier.

Many of the statistics quoted have been for men. It is true that in the younger age groups (thirty to forty years) men are more prone to heart disease than women and the surveys carried out and reported above are concerned mainly with men, e.g. the London busmen, the Institute of Directors survey and so on, but women too suffer from heart diseases and high blood cholesterol levels.

Traditionally, women have seemed to concern themselves with protecting their husbands' health, sometimes at the expense of their own. It is often the wife who encourages her husband to take regular exercise, to stop smoking, to have a regular medical check-up and generally to see that he keeps in good health. But women too produce cholesterol and suffer from arteriosclerosis and heart diseases. The main difference seems to be that the age when the symptoms develop appears to be about ten years later than for men.

There may be several reasons for this phenomenon. One is possibly the result of the menopause and its effect on sex hormones. Cholesterol is concerned in the production of hormones and it may be that during the menopause changes occur which affect the cholesterol levels in the blood. Another possibility is diet. More and more women seem to indulge in a form of slimming diet at some period in their life, often when they are younger, and weight reducing diets are often low in many of the foods that contribute saturated fats and cholesterol. All slimming diets involve a reduction in the total calorie intake and this in itself will result in the consumption of less food which can be converted by the body into cholesterol.

Once a woman suffers a heart attack the statistics show that it is likely to be more serious than for a male of similar age. One reason could be that a woman who suffers from coronary heart disease is likely to have an even higher cholesterol level than a male suffering from a similar condition. A woman with a cholesterol level over 270 is three times more likely to suffer a fatal attack than one whose level is below 270.

Although women are less likely to have a heart attack than men, after the mid-forties their arteries are becoming less healthy more quickly. Women with diabetes and high blood pressure are particularly prone to heart attacks, so if these conditions exist with a high cholesterol level they are very vulnerable to attack.

In 1981 the Department of Health and Social Security published a booklet *Avoiding Heart Attacks* in which preventative measures were discussed. The authors reviewed the arguments concerning ten factors which have been linked to the incidence of coronary heart disease. Three of these, cigarette smoking, hypertension and raised cholesterol levels, were given extra emphasis because they considered them to be of special importance. Each one of these in isolation, has a direct influence on the risk of developing coronary heart disease but when more than one is present the risk factor is increased.

High blood pressure and cigarette smoking can each be responsible for doubling the risk but together their influence is much more substantial. When high cholesterol levels are present in combination with raised blood pressure *and* smoking then, according to the D.H.S.S. booklet, the risk of coronary heart disease is up to eight times greater than for those without these high risk factors.

The risk factors are shown in the following table:

Characteristic:	Risk of Coronary Heart Disease:
Principal risk factors	
Cigarette smoking	The more smoked the greater the risk
Blood pressure	The higher the pressure the greater the risk
Blood cholesterol	The greater the concentration (especially of LDL – see Chapter 6) the greater the risk
Other factors	
Diabetes	Diabetics have a greater risk

Family history	Children of parents who do not suffer from coronary heart disease have a lower risk
Obesity	There may be a risk from being overweight
Stress	Possibly increases the risk
Personality	Some types may be more likely to develop heart disease than others
Physical activity	Regular exercise appears to reduce the risk
Hardness of water	There is some evidence that the softer the tap water the greater the risk.

Cholesterol, even if it is not all bad, is certainly dangerous. Diet, regular exercise, a reduction in the number of cigarettes smoked, can all help to avoid the undoubted risks of coronary heart disease and are to be encouraged even amongst the younger members of society. But there is another practical and positive step which can be taken. A daily supplement of pure soya lecithin can help to prevent the build-up of cholesterol and other fats in the arteries and also to reduce the levels already existing. It is easy to take and is a natural food. What is more, in many cases it will lead to an improvement in general health and physical and mental well-being.

5.

PROTECTING YOUR HEART

The human body has often been described as resembling a complex chemical plant needing a vast range of raw materials to maintain life and health. These chemical processes, which take place to convert the food we eat into energy or to build new cells or to perform all the other natural functions which occur, are happening twenty-four hours a day all through our lives. The body has its own highly sophisticated computer, the brain, which can only function if the correct type and amount of energy is provided by the diet. It carries out its own maintenance, and has a built-in warning system for when things go wrong. All this happens so quietly and efficiently that it goes unnoticed until something causes a disease to develop or an organ ceases to function normally. The principal bulk raw materials used by the body are proteins, fats and carbohydrates but, in order for these to be processed by the body, a large number of secondary materials are required. These are the vitamins, minerals, amino acids, enzymes, etc, and food must contain adequate quantities of all of them if the chemical reactions which take place in the body are to occur. The diet needs to be varied as much as possible so that a proper balance between the essential nutrients is achieved.

Diet has changed considerably in this century since civilized nations have become more affluent. As the people have become more wealthy they have demanded richer foods; as the pace of life increased they required easy to prepare convenience foods. Bigger markets have led increasingly to mass production of staple foods such as bread. This change in diet has led to an enormous increase in diseases that were rare, or even unknown, before 1900 and which are still virtually non-existent in more primitive communities. One result of this change in diet, especially in the industrialized nations of the world, is that too much of the wrong type of fat is consumed and the blood consequently contains too high a proportion of cholesterol and other fats and too little lecithin.

Excessive cholesterol and other dietary fats or lipids in the human blood is now acknowledged to be directly associated with the disease known as atherosclerosis, a principal cause of coronary heart disease and the biggest single cause of death in many countries of the world. In America and Scandinavia, in Australia, Germany and the United Kingdom, leading medical authorities all recognize that a reduction of blood cholesterol and other lipids is essential to protect the health of the nation. The old idea that atherosclerosis was an unavoidable result of growing old, or the effect of wear on the artery wall, has long since been abandoned. In Australia, a major meat producing nation, experiments are being conducted into feeding cattle with a diet rich in polyunsaturated fats so that the beef produced will be less harmful to the heart.

Reducing Cholesterol
There is strong evidence which shows that, in experimental animals, atherosclerosis can be reversed and there is evidence too that suggests the same is true in human beings. Modern treatment indicates that the reduction of blood cholesterol and lipids to normal levels is the best way to combat the symptoms of atherosclerosis. This has been achieved in two ways, the first of which is to modify the diet by reducing the amount of saturated fats and substituting polyunsaturated fats. In many cases this has not been easy to accomplish and the second method, the use of cholesterol lowering agents, has been tried. These have been mostly drugs and chemical substances which have been accepted only with misgivings, because of unwanted side-effects. These are particularly worrying since the drugs need to be used over a long period of time. What is required is a natural food product which can be incorporated into the diet and which will be valuable in both treating and preventing high blood cholesterol levels. Pure soya bean lecithin is such a product. To be effective it needs to be taken regularly and it must be a very biologically active form of lecithin. The type

recommended by all the leading nutritional authorities has a high phosphatidyl choline content, rich in poly-unsaturates and is available in granular form.

It appears that cholesterol and lecithin almost always exist side by side. When they are present in equilibrium lecithin is able to control cholesterol. It is only when an imbalance occurs that cholesterol takes over. In the bloodstream this results in arteriosclerosis; in the gall-bladder it leads to the formation of gallstones. The principal cause of imbalance is faulty diet, brought about by the conditions described at the beginning of this chapter.

I have previously described how cholesterol is deposited in the artery walls and how the emulsifying properties of lecithin are used by the body to prevent this occurring. In addition to being a very efficient emulsifier, lecithin also exhibits a number of other properties which influence its function within the human body. It plays an important part in fat metabolism, especially in the liver where most of the cholesterol is produced. It is incorporated into all the body tissues and has a vital role to play in the transport of lipids in the bloodstream.

Other cholesterol reducing agents are very different from lecithin. Under normal conditions they do not form part of the structure of blood fats, but lecithin is, of itself, a very necessary part of the mixture of fats and proteins which circulate in the blood. Lecithin is a phosphatide and as such is an essential stabilizing agent for the fat which circulates in the blood. When too much cholesterol and other fats are present in blood plasma they give a cloudy, milky appearance to the blood, but with the emulsifying properties available from lecithin, a clear solution is maintained. This is easily demonstrated, for when cholesterol is added to water it produces a cloudy, white mixture caused by the insoluble particles of fat, but if sufficient lecithin is added the cholesterol is dispersed as tiny particules instead of large lumps, and a clear solution results. This is what happens in the blood, enabling the cholesterol to pass through the artery walls and into the capillaries, the tiny vessels which carry blood to the body tissue.

Clearing the Arteries

The second problem in arteriosclerosis is the removal of cholesterol which has already been deposited. The cholesterol which is laid down in the arteries is in a solid form and in order for it to be solubilized it has to be converted into a form which can be washed off the artery wall by the vigorous action of the blood. This requires both the presence of lecithin as a phospholipid and polyunsaturated fatty acids. Scientists have demonstrated that a saturated lecithin, such as is obtained from egg yolk, is not effective in solubilizing cholesterol, whereas a polyunsaturated lecithin from soya greatly influences the transformation of cholesterol into a soluble form.

Cholesterol produced in the body dissolves at $149°C$, a very high temperature, but when it forms a compound with lecithin the resultant cholesterol lecithin complex dissolves at a temperature lower than normal body heat. This liquified cholesterol can then be washed off the artery wall. As it is removed it enters the blood stream, causing a temporary increase in the total amount of cholesterol in the blood. However, it is soon reduced and the levels begin to fall.

The consumption of polyunsaturated oils alone, that is without lecithin, would be insufficient to remove cholesterol. Only in the presence of lecithin can the essential fatty acids be effective in dissolving cholesterol. Because the majority of diets contain foods with a high proportion of saturated fats, there is a strong possibility that the lecithin produced in the liver will be a saturated type. That is why a soya lecithin supplement is so invaluable in the treatment and prevention of arteriosclerosis.

Experimental Evidence For Lecithin

One of the most important and enlightening experiments conducted into the ability of lecithin to reduce blood cholesterol levels in human beings was carried out by Dr Lester Morrison, the Director of a research unit at the Los Angeles County General Hospital. Dr Morrison selected twenty-one patients who had been in his care for one or ten years. All had been treated with cholesterol reducing agents other than lecithin and all had been on a specially prescribed low fat diet, so that the blood cholesterol levels were comparatively fixed. All had high blood cholesterol counts and one woman patient was as high as 1012 milligrammes per 100 millilitres of blood serum. Six patients did not complete the tests which ran for three months. In twelve of the remaining fifteen cases very significant falls in the level of cholesterol were noted. The average fall in the patients responding to the lecithin treatment was a remarkable 156 milligrammes or 41 per cent. Dr Morrison concluded his report by stating that lecithin was found to be the most effective cholesterol reducing agent tested to date.

The lecithin chosen for this trial was a pure granular form of soya lecithin containing over 90 per cent of natural phospholipids. Dr Morrison in his report, draws attention to the fact that, although the cholesterol lowering effects of soya bean lecithin had been demonstrated in previous studies, the products used had a high proportion of soya bean oil and there was uncertainty therefore as to whether the polyunsaturates in the oil had contributed an unknown factor. The pure lecithin used contained only a negligible amount of soya oil and the striking results obtained were entirely due to the lecithin. Pure lecithin granules are now on sale in many countries throughout the world.

They can be purchased in the United Kingdom from all health food stores. There are several brands available but it is most important that the one you select contains only pure lecithin granules. Some products contain lecithin mixed with milk powder or soya flour and there are now some granules on sale which contain fruit and other flavours. All these types of products are helpful but in order to obtain the full benefit from pure lecithin you are advised to consult the retailer who will recommend the most suitable product for you to take.

Other prominent scientists and nutritional experts support the view that lecithin (or phospholipids) in the blood offer protection from coronary heart disease. An article entitled 'Assessing the Coronary Profile' in the American journal *Geriatrics* observed that increased phospholipids may be a protective factor in coronary heart disease and may modify the significance of raised concentrations of cholesterol in the blood. Another writer in the *Journal of Nutrition* describes how a patient with a cholesterol count over 1000 was able to drop to 182 after taking soya lecithin for three months. Adelle Davis in her well-known books also has a lot to say about the ability of lecithin to influence blood cholesterol levels.

During the last twenty years there has been an enormous amount of scientific interest in the relationship between cholesterol and heart disease and how the diet and nutritional supplements can help to prevent the build-up of cholesterol in the blood. It is now almost universally accepted that there is direct link, and this can be seen from many scientific papers which have been published reporting on experiments in both animals and humans as well as population studies. It has become clear that there is a direct link between the level of cholesterol and the risk from coronary heart disease.

During the last few years scientists have not been so much concerned as to whether cholesterol was responsible, but how and why the factors which increase the risk of coronary heart disease occur. This has meant an enormous increase in the amount of interest in cholesterol and the different forms in which it occurs within the body and a later chapter reports on the most recent developments.

Blood Clots

There is another major cause of fatal heart disease, coronary thrombosis. In atherosclerosis the artery is blocked by fatty substances which eventually, after a number of years, completely block the passage and interrupt the flow of blood to the heart, causing in many cases a fatal attack. A thrombosis, however, is caused by a clot occurring in the blood. If this is large enough to prevent the flow of blood back to the heart it again causes a heart attack. Whatever the cause of the restriction within the coronary artery, if the circulation is cut off, a fatal heart attack may occur. If the blockage is not complete and the circulation is restricted sufficiently to reduce the oxygen reaching the heart, then the pain known as angina occurs.

Clots are formed when the blood cells called platelets become 'sticky', causing them to mass together to form a lump. This happens when excessive blood fats, rather than cholesterol, are present and can occur even when atherosclerosis is not in an advanced state. The more saturated fat in the blood, the greater the risk of clotting. Whenever the diet contains a large amount of saturated fat there is a high rate of death from coronary thrombosis. Obviously, if atherosclerosis is present there is a greater risk of a clot blocking the circulation completely because the arteries have been made narrower, but thrombosis can occur even without excess cholesterol. The evidence available suggests that people suffering from thrombosis lack the nutrients required to utilize fats, and the essential nutrient that can help to prevent clots forming is lecithin.

In people prone to heart disease the particles of fat in the blood are large. In a healthy individual they circulate as tiny droplets which can pass through the artery walls. Large particles of fat can act as a barrier on which sticky platelets collect and, by reducing circulation, cause blood cells to form into clots. Lecithin, as previously explained, acts as an emulsifier, breaking down fat into tiny particles and holding them in suspension, so that by breaking down these small particles, it removes the restrictions which can encourage the formation of clots. Numerous experiments and observations have shown that in patients who suffer from coronary heart disease blood lecithin has consistently been low, and the lower the level the greater the risk of clotting.

The adhesiveness of the platelets, which form into clots, has been shown to be affected by the amount of polyunsaturated fatty acids available in the diet. The mechanism by which this takes place is not fully understood, for not all the polyunsaturates have the same ability to reduce the clotting time of blood. When subjects are given soya oil or linseed oil there is a marked reduction in the stickiness of the platelets; but when other polyunsaturated oils, such as corn or safflower oil, are given the result is less apparent. This is probably because the first two are richer in linolenic acid, the rarest of the polyunsaturates, whilst the other two are rich in essential linoleic acid. Pure soya lecithin contains both these essential fatty acids and this probably accounts for its ability to help in both atherosclerosis and coronary thrombosis.

Dietary Dangers

Sugar is often thought to be another major dietary cause of heart disease. This is not surprising since it is a well-known fact that this particular carbohydrate is easily converted by the body into the type of fat known as 'triglycerides'. Some of these inevitably find their way into the blood stream along with the other fats. The same thing happens when alcohol and many refined foods are consumed and consequently the risk of heart disease developing is increased.

There is an argument which often develops between nutritional authorities as to which is the principal dietary cause of heart attacks, cholesterol or the other fats, the triglycerides. Why, for instance, do Eskimos in Greenland develop heart attacks when those in Alaska, who have accepted an American style diet, have the same risk factor as the rest of the population? The traditional Eskimo diet consists largely of marine fat and has little or no refined carbohydrate such as alcohol or sugar. The polyunsaturates in the high-fat fish diet probably account for this, for although the blood may contain cholesterol the level of triglycerides formed from carbohydrate is low. The incidence of heart disease around the shores of the Mediterranean Sea is also low. Traditional diets in this region are high in unrefined or 'virgin' olive oil which, although low in polyunsaturates, does contain the phospholipids (lecithin) removed from the refined oil sold in other countries. The Japanese in Japan have a low rate of heart disease but those living in America, who have accepted the American way of life and diet, have the same high risk rate as the average American. The Japanese diet obtains only about 3 per cent of calories from saturated fats and this is almost certainly why the rate of heart disease is low. The significance of this is that whatever the cause – whether it be high cholesterol or triglycerides in the blood, too much of the wrong fat has a serious adverse effect on the heart and in each case lecithin, the fat fighter, can help to keep the level down.

Vitamins Which Help The Heart

Although lecithin is so important in the control of cholesterol, other nutrients can also keep the heart healthy. Many nutrients contribute to health and they are all interdependent. Vitamins, for example, have many roles to play in both the treatment and prevention of disease. It is not perhaps surprising that the fat-soluble vitamins A and E influence fat metabolism, but so also do vitamin C and the B complex. A recent article in *The Lancet* reported that garlic could lower blood cholesterol – almost certainly because it is a powerful anti-oxidant and serves to prevent oxidation of the polyunsaturates in the body.

Vitamin E

The work of the famous Drs Shute in Canada is well known through the world and vitamin E is now taken by hundreds of people to protect their heart against disease. According to the Shute brothers, vitamin E acts in several ways to influence the overall health of the heart, the most important of which are listed here.

(a) It increases the ability of the circulatory system to carry blood and oxygen to the heart and limits the heart's requirement of oxygen.

(b) Vitamin E acts as a natural anti-clotting agent. It does not interfere with normal clotting of blood in a wound, but it does seem to help stop the platelets in the arteries from forming into clots.

(c) It is best known for its anti-oxidant properties which help to protect polyunsaturated acids, which are so easily oxidized, from turning rancid.

(d) Vitamin E appears to exert a strengthening action on the capillaries, those tiny blood vessels which are so easily damaged; and, when they have been damaged, it helps to rebuild them.

(e) After a thrombosis has occurred vitamin E helps to keep damaged tissue soft and flexible.

Soya lecithin contains its own natural store of precious vitamin E, but extra supplies can be obtained from health stores in the form of capsules. It is important always to choose the right supplement and the best and easily the most potent is natual vitamin E, called d'alpha tocopherol, which is 36 per cent more active than its synthetic counterpart.

Vitamin B Complex
All the vitamins in the B group seem to be used in the metabolism of fats, but the most important in this connection are choline and inositol. These two little known vitamins also occur naturally in soya lecithin, and in the pure granular form of lecithin they are present in large amounts linked with the phospholipids. Choline and inositol are necessary nutrients for the body, they enable the liver to produce its own lecithin. Both these vitamins have been reported to be useful in lowering blood cholesterol levels. One teaspoonful of soya lecithin granules will contain approximately 115 mg each of choline and inositol. Since all the vitamins in the B group are interrelated it is always advisable to take a supplement which contains all the important B Complex vitamins in a single capsule or tablet.

Vitamin A
Dr Lester Morrison, who has already been mentioned for his work with lecithin in the reduction of blood cholesterol levels, recommends vitamin A in his book *The Low Fat Way to Health and Longer Life* and, in *Let's Get Well*, Adelle Davis tells of medical reports describing how vitamin A helped heart patients. Apparently after large doses of this vitamin had been given daily for three to six months, cholesterol levels fell and the lecithin in the blood increased.

The natural sources of vitamin A are carrots, leafy vegetables and fish liver oils. Once again, very good supplements are available and can be purchased from health stores.

Vitamin C

Another natural anti-oxidant, vitamin C, has also been shown to help reduce blood cholesterol levels. Dr Spittle writing in *The Lancet* reports that vitamin C can help reduce the accumulation of cholesterol deposits in the artery walls, by loosening them so that they can be washed out of the system. She also tells of other tests where one experimental group was given a high fat diet with no vitamin C and the other the same high fat diet but with large doses of vitamin C. The first group developed symptoms of heart disease, but the second group did not develop heart trouble.

Bran

Primitive tribes such as the Masai in Africa appear relatively free from heart troubles, even though their diet is high in saturated fats. Many researchers believe that this is because the diet is high in natural fibre. Bran is a dietary fibre which has been shown to have many beneficial functions in the treatment of the diseases of civilization. It is an excellent natural laxative which helps to remove surplus cholesterol from the body. It also provides a good supply of B vitamins.

Heart diseases can be caused by other influences which have not been considered in this book, such as cigarette smoking, obesity, lack of exercise. Diabetics and persons suffering from high blood pressure also carry a high risk factor. What has been attempted here is to point out that one very important factor in the increasing rate of death from heart disease is faulty diet. Diets that encourage high levels of cholesterol and other fats in the blood are without any doubt responsible for a large number of unnecessary deaths from heart disease. Changes in the type and amount of food consumed are essential, but since atherosclerosis is a condition that takes years to develop to the point where it exercises a noticeable adverse effect on the heart, a change in diet cannot be expected to reverse the problem overnight. There exists, however, sufficient evidence to indicate that one nutrient, soya lecithin, can and does help to reduce cholesterol and other blood fats to an acceptable level. It is not claimed to be a miracle worker, just a natural food which modern diet has neglected or destroyed and which has a very important job to do in protecting the health of that most vital organ – the heart.

Other Dietary Methods of Influencing Heart Disease

In America much more importance has been given to dietary methods of influencing heart disease than in the U.K. In fact *Doctor* magazine in April 1982 reported that Dr William Kennel, in a study sponsored by the American Heart Association, claimed that British doctors are apathetic about giving advice on dietary control of heart disease. He said that British doctors were sceptical about the benefits of how changes in the diet affect heart disease and are slow to suggest that we should cut down the amount of fat we eat. In America much dietary advice has been given both by consumer bodies and by Government sponsored reports and the result of this is that deaths from heart disease among Americans have been falling quite rapidly and over the last few years there has been a 25 per cent decline in heart disease deaths in America. Reduced smoking and more exercise together with changes in diet, particularly the switch from saturated fats to polyunsaturated fats, have undoubtedly contributed to this improvement.

In Britain, the Coronary Prevention Group have called on doctors to recommend to their patients a number of simple steps that can be taken to improve their health. The most important of these are:

1. Many of us are overweight and a reduction in weight can improve the health of the heart.

2. Exercise should be encouraged to prevent the risk of heart disease.

3. Excessive use of salt should be cut down. This can lead to high blood pressure which in turn can increase the risk of heart disease.

4. Fat in the diet should be reduced but not at the expense of valuable polyunsaturated fats.

5. Foods with high dietary fibre should be increased.

6. Children need special attention because dietary habits are established early, and if a good diet can be adopted early in life the habit remains.

In addition to the above it is also quite clear that smoking is a very high contributory factor in coronary heart disease.

If some or all of the above methods were adopted throughout the population then, undoubtedly, we could make the same strides to reduce the incidence of heart disease as have already been made in America.

6.
THE NEW RESEARCH ON CHOLESTEROL

By the mid 1970s it had become clear to medical scientists and biochemists that there was a very positive link between cholesterol and heart disease. This had been borne out in both animal and human experiments and by long-term population studies. In order to explain why vegetable oils had a cholesterol lowering effect while animal fats had the reverse, further research was obviously necessary. It had also been noticed that although lecithin and vegetable oils both contain high proportions of polyunsaturated fats, especially linoleic acid, lecithin seemed to be more beneficial in both its cholesterol lowering properties and its ability to protect the heart.

We know that fats are transported around the body in the bloodstream. Amongst these fats are lecithin and cholesterol and they are carried round in the blood with proteins, which are fat and protein mixtures. When these proteins, which are fat and protein mixtures. When the lipo-proteins are examined it is found that they fall into two different categories, some of the have got a very low density, and some of them have a much higher density. Scientists call them low density lipo-proteins (LDL) and high density lipo-proteins (HDL) and research has concentrated on the difference between these two types of lipo-protein.

Low density lipo-proteins carry about 70 per cent of blood cholesterol while high density lipo-proteins carry about 15 per cent (there are other types of lipo-proteins but these two are by far the most significant). Could it be that one of them was more responsible for the build-up of cholesterol on artery walls and, if so, could the differences between the proportions of LDL and HDL in the blood be related in any way to the incidence of heart disease? This was the question that needed to be answered.

It was noticed by an American biochemist that while dogs never get atherosclerosis, rabbits, when fed a diet rich in saturated fats, quickly develop this complaint. What causes the dog to have a natural protection when the rabbit doesn't? Dr Kritchevsky explains the difference in terms of LDL and HDL. Dogs apparently have got a very high proportion of HDL cholesterol compared with their LDL cholesterol. So great is the difference that it is almost impossible to induce atherosclerosis in dogs however the diet is varied, but the same is not true for rabbits who develop it quickly. Rabbits have about equal proportions of HDL and LDL. Could this be a significant factor in the protection from coronary heart disease? Apparently it can. Studies in humans have indicated that where HDL is high in relation to LDL there are significantly less artery problems and a lower incidence of heart disease.

The Israel Ischaemic Heart Disease Study examined deaths from coronary heart disease over a seven year period. They discovered that when less than 14 per cent of the total cholesterol in the blood was carried as HDL there were 29 deaths per 1,000. Where more than 23 per cent of total cholesterol was carried as HDL this dropped to 4 deaths per 1,000 and their findings are illustrated in the table below.

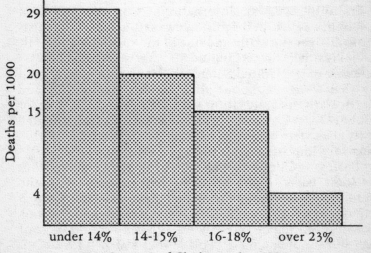

Per Centage of Cholesterol as HDL

This is just one of the many studies which have been published in the last few years which indicate that there is a very real link between HDL and LDL and it is now recognized that where LDL is high there is an increased risk of coronary heart disease and where HDL is high there is less risk, and this is well supported by statistical studies. Somehow HDL picks up cholesterol and transfers it to the liver where it is metabolized and excreted in bile acids. So where there is plenty of HDL in the blood there is less risk of coronary heart disease.

These findings are also supported by examination of the blood of athletes. It would appear that when regular exercise is taken there is less risk of heart disease and athletes tend to have much higher levels of HDL in their blood than non-athletes.

It now becomes obvious that, although it is important to lower blood cholesterol levels, it is not just a question of total cholesterol being reduced. It is far more important that the type of cholesterol which is lowered is that carried by LDL and if cholesterol can be lowered at the same time that LDL is lowered and HDL is increased or maintained, so that the proportion of HDL to LDL is increased, then there is far less risk of coronary heart disease.

In April 1982 an International Congress on Soya Lecithin was held at Brighton. It was attended by scientists from all over the world and one of the sponsors was G. R. Lane Health Products Limited who market *Lecigran Lecithin Granules* in the United Kingdom. Many papers were read at this Congress about the benefits of lecithin and particularly its association with HDL and LDL. Doctor Howard from Cambridge said that while all polyunsaturated fatty acids were beneficial in lowering cholesterol, lecithin was very important because of its effect on HDL.

Professor Cairella from Rome University reported that in some parts of the world he had observed that the amount of lecithin in the diet had dropped from 3 grams per day to less than 0.7 grams per day and that this was not sufficient. He underlined the importance of lecithin supplements to replace that which is lost.

One of the most important papers read at the Conference

was by Professor Hawthorn and his co-workers from Nottingham University. He stated that it was the quality of polyunsaturated fats that was important in considering their ability to remove cholesterol from the body and that soya bean lecithin was the most effective type of poly-unsaturated fatty acids. He backed up his statement with results of research being conducted at the University Medical School. Trials in both rats and humans had indicated that when the polyunsaturated fatty acid linoleic acid was fed as lecithin, it had a far better effect on the levels of HDL than when a corresponding amount was fed of vegetable oil. In a two week trial on normal humans total cholesterol was reduced by 2.6 per cent, but the level of HDL increased by 8.9 per cent and LDL cholesterol was lowered by 7.3 per cent. In a four week period the cholesterol level fell by 5.8 per cent and although the HDL and LDL were both lowered there was a much greater lowering of LDL. Lecithin had not just reduced cholesterol but it had improved the balance between HDL and LDL in favour of HDL and this would indicate, from the evidence available, that it would help to protect against heart disease. He also reported on trials designed to show that HDL plays an important part in the removal of cholesterol from the body and explained how it transferred it to the liver for excretion in the form of bile acids.

Although the pathway by which lecithin is able to influence the levels of HDL is understood, it is still not clear how this happens, only that the cholesterol is removed from the body. Obviously further work has still to be done to enable us to fully understand the implications of the current research.

An article in the magazine *Athero-sclerosis* in 1981 reported on a six weeks trial using corn oil which produced little change in HDL cholesterol level, while the corresponding trial for six weeks using lecithin instead of corn oil increased the HDL and lowered the LDL, and many other papers have indicated similar findings. The recent research is important because it tells us not just that lecithin can lower cholesterol but begins to explain how it happens. It does, however, make it much more difficult to understand and it may be useful therefore to summarise the situation.

Cholesterol in the blood is carried either as low density or high density lipo-proteins. Studies of populations and trends over the past few years have shown that increased concentrations of low density lipo-protein (LDL) are harmful in relation to heart disease. On the other hand HDL has a beneficial role to play in cholesterol removal. Where there are high LDL cholesterol levels or low HDL cholesterol levels the risk factor for man is high and it is advisable to lower LDL cholesterol while at the same time increasing or maintaining the levels of HDL so that there is an increase in the HDL/LDL ratio.

Professor Assmann of West Germany, speaking at the Brighton Conference, stated that, with improved methods of analysis in the measurement of HDL and new statistical information, in the future we shall be able to predict more precisely those people at risk from coronary heart disease.

Recent British statistics on deaths from heart disease when compared with those from America and other countries such as Australia, Canada and Finland indicate that we have not made as much progress as these other countries in controlling mortality rates. At best, the rates in Britain are only flattening out, while in other countries, particularly the United States, they are falling. We must accept that there is not yet rigorous proof of the benefit of preventative medicine and changes in diet but there is certainly enough circumstantial evidence to suggest that the positive steps that have been outlined, and particularly the advisability of taking a regular lecithin supplement, may indeed be very beneficial.

7.
STAYING SLIM AND HEALTHY

Lecithin has been described as a most versatile nutrient concerned with the metabolism of fat within the human body. This means that it has many important functions in addition to offering protection from the heart. When a clot of blood forms in a coronary artery it can cause a heart attack, but thrombosis can occur in other arteries and veins and many cause phlebitis, varicose veins or a stroke. The way in which these occur is similar to that described in Chapter 5 and lecithin can exert a similar influence to protect the body from the consequences. Fat and cholesterol are responsible for other threats to good health, and this chapter describes some of them, telling how and why lecithin can assist the body to overcome them.

Lecithin for Weight Reduction

Although it is perhaps an oversimplification to suggest that they are the only reasons, there are two main motives for wanting to slim. The first and most common is concerned with appearance and the desire (amongst men as well as women) to have a trim figure, free from unsightly bulges. The second reason is that excessive weight is damaging to good health. There are thousands of words written every week in books and women's magazines offering specialist advice to the would-be slimmer. Special diets and exercise plans abound, health farms and other aids exist in profusion – and so much so that the cynic often remarks that there is only one real way to slim and that is to eat less food. While it is almost universally true that we eat too much, diet is far too critical to health to be treated so lightly and slimming régimes need to be approached with great care, otherwise the diet may be deficient in one or more of the essential nutrients. Whatever the reason for slimming, be it obesity or to improve the figure, lecithin, the fat fighter, can help.

Many tablets and charts exist which show the 'average' body weight which is desirable for a given height and age. These are of little use to the individual except as a very rough guide. All of us are individuals and subject to a different body structure. Bone and muscle contribute to weight as do fat and excess fluid, but generally speaking it is the fat and fluid which produce the unsightly bulges that most slimmers strive so hard to lose. Depot fat stored throughout the body and particularly around the waist, thighs and upper arms is the fat which needs to be removed in order to shed the plumpness that so many people attempt to lose with their slimming diets.

The type of fat which makes us appear to be fat is not necessarily the result of eating too much fatty food. All food contributes energy which is measured in calories. If we consume more calories than we burn up as energy then the surplus is converted by the body into depot fat, which is stored under the skin until it is required for energy production. This type of fat is not only provided by fatty foods. Protein and carbohydrates are easily converted by the body into fat, which is why sugar and other refined carbohydrates such as alcohol and starches are restricted in many diets. Provided that the body is functioning normally, then a diet which restricts the number of calories eaten will help to reduce weight by forcing the body to draw on its store of depot fat to provide energy.

Lecithin is the nutrient which has a major function in assisting the body to burn up fat. Although it is itself a fat and contributes some calories, its value in utilizing other fats far outweighs its addition to the total number of calories consumed. This is because soya lecithin is a phospholipid which is partly absorbed intact and not used for the production of energy in the way in which other fats, carbohydrates and proteins are. Lecithin burns up fat faster than any other nutrient and its addition to a slimming diet will greatly assist in weight reduction, always remembering that calorie control is carried out.

The second way that lecithin can help to get rid of those extra inches is by keeping the fats on the move. Lecithin is a biological emulsifier; in the manufacture of chocolate it is used to keep the product mobile and flowing. It does the same to the fat in your body: keeps moving it around so that it cannot form deposits in unwanted places. By keeping the fat broken down into small particles, lecithin ensures that it is burned up more thoroughly and quickly by the body, using all the nutrients from the fat and preventing it being stored.

Adelle Davis tells of one investigation where people on a 500 calorie a day diet of carbohydrate lost no weight but when they received five times that number of calories from protein and fat (including oil which contained the ingredients necessary for the body to produce lecithin) they lost weight. Equally important was the observation that those who lost weight with oil in the diet did not put weight back on once they had reached the desired weight, providing oil was still present in the diet. Vegetable oils enable the body to build lecithin, but a more certain way is to take a lecithin supplement as part of a weight reducing campaign, whatever régime is followed.

The third way that lecithin can help is by preventing the retention of water within the body, for although it is only water it looks just like fat and makes the individual who has a water-retention problem feel fat. Lecithin is a natural diuretic, that is, it helps to remove excess fluid from the system and while this fluid may not form a significant amount of the total body weight, fluid can cause bulges which are just as unsightly as those caused by fat.

Three good reasons, then, why lecithin can help the slimmer to reduce weight and improve the shape. Whichever type of diet is favoured, low calorie or low carbohydrate, the action of lecithin on fat in the body is equally important in achieving the desired results and, because it is a natural food, it is safe to use. When dieting, for whatever reason, it must be remembered that a balanced diet is essential to maintain good health. Do not attempt to drastically reduce weight too quickly. A slow sure way will have a much better chance of success, with less risk of harm to general health and vitality. Make sure the essential vitamins and minerals are present in the food eaten, or else take a daily supplement to replace those lost by reducing the food intake. It pays dividends in the long-term.

Not all problems of weight are caused or corrected by the calorie content of food. Sometimes the body's inability to metabolize fat properly is the reason for an increase in body weight. In many cases lecithin can correct these problems which may be due to under-production of lecithin, and lecithin complexes with other nutrients, by the liver, so that fat is not burned up properly. Lecithin assists the body by making sure that fat can be properly utilized to produce energy requirements. If it is, then it cannot be stored within the tissues to create the lumps and bumps which the slimmer needs to lose.

Finally, in this section on weight, a word of warning to those fortunate people who are slim. Some lucky individuals never seem to vary in weight – they can eat as much as they like of whatever food they fancy, without adding to their store of depot fat. For them there are never problems of extra inches around the waist and consequently they eat as much food as they desire. They never need to diet and can eat butter, cream, fatty foods, carbohydrates such as sugar and alcohol and still they stay slim. Because of this they perhaps forget that the unseen fats are more dangerous even than the fats which can be seen. The foods they eat are probably rich in cholesterol and other dietary fats which find their way into the blood stream where they can produce arteriosclerosis and heart disease. Just because fat is not stored in the tissue, they ignore other problems associated with fat disorders caused by a diet rich in saturated fats and carbohydrates. For them, lecithin can offer its protective influence just as effectively.

Lecithin for the Liver

It is in the liver, the largest organ in the body, that a great many of the chemical processes necessary to maintain the health and well-being of the human body take place. It has been estimated that several thousand chemical reactions take place in the liver every second. Carbohydrates, proteins and fats are changed by the liver into sugars, starches and fats capable of being used by the body. It stores some of the vitamins, minerals and trace elements until they are needed and renders harmless such substances as drugs, poisons, and chemicals. Innumerable amino acids, enzymes and coenzymes are produced in the liver so that they can be used in other parts of the body to set up further essential chemical processes. The liver also produces lecithin, cholesterol, bile and blood albumen. All these functions and many others are performed by a healthy liver, providing all the essential nutrients that it needs are present in the diet. If the liver is damaged, or if the nutrients are not available, then the organ cannot function normally.

If the liver cannot utilize foods efficiently, either because of damage or nutritional deficiency, general symptoms of ill health will occur. For instance, insufficient bile may be produced, causing severe indigestion; or glycogen, which is a body starch made in the liver from sugar, cannot be produced or stored, leading to fatigue and overweight. An unhealthy liver cannot produce lecithin or metabolize fats properly.

One problem which occurs when the liver fails to synthesize sufficient lecithin is the condition known as fatty liver. Without sufficient lecithin those other body fats, the triglycerides, are not carried away from the liver and fatty deposits are formed. The cells become blocked, swollen and inflamed and become filled with fat that some of it finds its way into the blood and bile, especially when too much saturated fat is present. During stress due to widely varying reasons, the liver often reacts by laying down considerable quantities of fats in its tissue. This too gives rise to fatty liver.

A nutritional supplement of soya lecithin will assist in transporting these accumulated triglycerides away from the liver and, by providing choline and inositol, will furnish two of the essential building blocks needed by the liver to produce its own lecithin. When rats are fed on a diet deficient in choline, fat soon starts to accumulate in the liver. When choline is added to the diet the fat disperses and the liver returns to normal health. If liver cells are damaged scar tissue forms and a condition similar to cirrhosis of the liver occurs.

When the source of choline is lecithin the improvement

of the health of the liver is usually much faster, as part of the lecithin is absorbed directly by the liver and choline by itself is sometimes destroyed by bacteria present in the intestine. Not only can lecithin help fight liver disease, it is also especially important because it can protect against disorders of the liver. Lecithin plays a vital role within the liver and because so many bodily functions start within this organ it is important to maintain lecithin, either by making sure that a well-balanced diet provides all the necessary nutrients for the liver to produce its own supply or by regularly taking a lecithin supplement.

Dissolving Gallstones

The gall-bladder contains bile, a compound necessary to digest fats and to carry nutrients, such as the oil soluble vitamins A, D, E and K, into the blood. Bile contains three principal components, bile acids, lecithin and cholesterol, together with pigments. Apparently the lecithin has two separate functions, the first concerned with the metabolism of fat, the second its ability to control cholesterol.

Lecithin in the bile exerts an emulsifying action on the particles of fat, breaking them down into tiny droplets so that they can be digested by the enzymes and absorbed, enabling the body to utilize the fat.

It appears that the pigments and cholesterol are merely waste products and are excreted. However, cholesterol is a very hard type of fat, practically insoluble in water and the bile relies upon lecithin to hold the cholesterol in suspension. When the balance of lecithin-cholesterol-bile acids is disturbed, gallstones are formed which consist in the main of precipitated cholesterol. It is, therefore, important to maintain a high proportion of lecithin in the bile to prevent the formation of gall-stones.

Tests carried out by Dr D. M. Small at Boston University concerned the solubility of cholesterol gallstones. Bile salts alone were insufficient to dissolve these accumulations, whereas the solubility was much greater with a bile salt/phosphatidylcholine mixture. Granular soya lecithin contains a high proportion of this particular phospholipid. While these tests do not necessarily indicate that gallstones can be dissolved within the human body, it is certain that maintaining a high level of lecithin in the bile will help to prevent stones from forming and may reduce those which exist so that they can be eliminated from the system.

Diabetic Diets

In diabetes secondary symptoms generally occur, e.g. fatty deposits in the liver, metabolic disorders (such as those causing an increase in the fat and cholesterol levels in the blood) and changes in the blood vessels with arteriosclerotic symptoms. Lecithin has a direct influence on the reduction of these symptoms due to the part it plays in the metabolism of the liver and of fats. Above and beyond this, lecithin, with its high energy content, is a valuable source of energy for diabetics since it does not have the disadvantages of normal fats and carbohydrates.

Lecithin for the Nerves and Brain

The nerves and brain contain a large amount of lecithin. It has been calculated that the dry weight of the brain has 25 per cent lecithin, about twice the amount found in internal organs. The main part is used in the structure of cells and since the cells are constantly being rebuilt a regular supply of lecithin is essential.

Under stress conditions lecithin serves as a source of energy. Normally the brain derives its energy from glucose in the body but it has been shown that when stress conditions are induced the lecithin reserves decline significantly. This suggests that lecithin is being used as an additional source of energy, probably because it is activated more quickly than depot fat.

Although the brain can synthesize lecithin, it has been proved that some dietary lecithin is directly transported to the brain via the blood stream. Lecithin is, therefore, an important food both for the brain and the nerves, providing a readily usable source of energy in times of stress and, by helping to build nerve tissue, it can help relieve the problems caused by nerve damage. 'Shattered nerves', irritability, insomnia, lack of patience, are typical modern-day symptoms of tired, worn nerves. They are often the result of dietary deficiencies which can be corrected by either vitamin B complex supplements or by lecithin.

In multiple sclerosis, autopsies have shown decreased levels of lecithin in the brain and in the myelin sheath which covers and protects the nerves. Furthermore, the lecithin that is present contains a high proportion of saturated rather than polyunsaturated fatty acids. Population studies have shown that where the diet contains a high proportion of saturated fats then the incidence of multiple sclerosis is high, probably because blood lecithin is lower.

Multiple sclerosis can become more severe when there is a lack of any nutrient that assists lecithin production. Fewer bad periods have occurred when the diet has contained oils which stimulate lecithin production, or better still when a lecithin supplement has been given. No major research programme has yet been successfully conducted but experiments are now taking place in various centres, in an attempt to correct the severity of attacks of multiple sclerosis by dietary methods.

A Real Tonic!
In Germany lecithin is consumed in vast quantities for its tonic properties. Scientific studies have shown that high performance athletes recover more quickly after effort when lecithin is taken regularly. The same is true of individuals performing hard physical work and, because lecithin provides energy which can be absorbed directly by the brain, after mental exertion.

By improving the absorption of fats and by providing a good source of non-fattening energy, lecithin is a valuable food for convalescents and those on restricted diets. One of the observations made by Lester Morrison, in the report on his famous work in reducing blood cholesterol levels with lecithin, was that his patients frequently expressed the feeling that they felt better. They had more energy for both physical and mental exertion and their bowel function was often improved when taking the lecithin supplement.

8.
LECITHIN AND THE BRAIN

The brain is one of the most sensitive and vital organs of the body. It is also the least understood and although there has been a tremendous improvement in our knowledge of how the brain functions it is shrouded in mystery. Scientists have known for a long time that the brain requires a continuous source of oxygen and glucose and that if anything interferes with the supply of these two nutrients then irreversible brain damage will be caused within minutes. Because the brain is so vital to the functioning of the whole body it has its own inbuilt mechanisms for regulating the flow of blood and the nutrients which blood supplies. The brain controls the flow of substances from the blood enabling it to synthesize compounds according to its needs at a particular time.

For many years scientists believed that something they called the blood-brain barrier protected the brain from the effects of nutrients which were either deficient or excessive in the daily diet. They knew of only a very few things, principally alcohol and powerful drugs, which were thought to be able to breach the blood-brain barrier and directly affect the brain. In the mid 1970s nutritional researchers began to discover that, in a few instances, what a person eats can and does have direct influence on how the brain works and therefore how that person behaves. Much of the new research stems from the work of Dr William J. Wurtman and his colleagues in the Department of Nutrition and Food Science at the Massachusetts Institute of Technology. Dr Wurtman and his fellow researchers have clear evidence that among the few substances which can break through the blood-brain barrier is choline and the finest dietary source of choline is, of course, lecithin. Referring to the ability of choline to affect the brain, Dr Wurtman comments in *Chemical and Engineering News* 'this is an extraordinary way for the brain to work. Until we did this work, everybody, myself included, would have told you that the brain regulates its own business. That the brain is so important that it gets whatever it needs from the circulation. If heat is in short supply, warm blood goes there and the cold blood to the periphery. If glucose is in short supply the glucose goes there, or oxygen, or whatever is needed. So the brain, by virtue of this exalted position, has been thought to be immune to whatever was taking place in the rest of the body.'

The work of Dr Wurtman and his colleagues has shown that there is a direct connection between the food we eat and the way the brain works. In effect diet can and does influence the functioning of the brain.

The substances in the brain which respond to dietary choline are called neurotransmitters. The human brain contains billions of neurons. These minute cells control all aspect of behaviour including thought, speech, mood, memory, sensation and mobility. The neurotransmitters are chemical signals, like electric impulses, which conduct information through the nervous system from one neuron to another, or to muscle or other cells. We know of about thirty neurotransmitters and there are probably others still to be discovered. Exactly how many exist and what function each helps to control is not yet clear. The neurotransmitters are synthesized in the brain cells and during the past few years it has been discovered that choline in the brain influences the rate at which one of the neurotransmitters, acetylcholine, is produced. The choline which passes through the blood-brain barrier is obtained from one of two sources. It is either produced by the liver or is obtained from dietary sources, mainly in the form of lecithin. Dr Wurtman and others have shown that dietary supplementation of choline increases the brain level and the amount of acetylcholine the brain is able to produce. Furthermore, when choline was taken in its natural form as lecithin, it was even more effective in raising the blood choline levels in humans.

The discovery that a common dietary substance, lecithin, had an almost immediate effect on the brain function excited scientists all over the world and since the late 1970s has prompted wide-spread research. Promising results have been obtained in treating one disabling brain disorder and research into others is continuing to find out if lecithin can improve memory, or depression, senile dementia and other abnormalities, caused by a deficiency of the neurotransmitter, acetylcholine, in the brain.

Many researchers prefer treating their patients with lecithin rather than the drug choline chloride. This is because not only has it been shown that lecithin is more effective at raising blood levels of choline, it is also free of side-effects associated with the drug. One side-effect is that people who take the drug in large and regular doses develop an odour of rotten fish and this is avoided when lecithin is taken!

One of the most dramatic results which has arisen from the recent discoveries is in the treatment of a fairly common disorder called Tardive Dyskinesia. This is a condition which develops in mental patients who are regularly treated with very powerful drugs which are used to calm the patients and to give them relief from the acute symptoms of their mental illness. After long periods of time taking these drugs, patients often develop involuntary twitches of the tongue and muscles of the mouth, which make speech very difficult, and they often develop uncontrollable jerky movements of the upper body and limbs. These are extremely distressing and unpleasant symptoms and for a person already handicapped by the problems of mental illness the symptoms can be psychologically devastating. Some estimates are that up to 40 per cent of elderly long-term psychiatric patients may suffer from this illness and it is often so severe that it limits the use of drugs necessary to treat the original illness.

Several drugs have been used to treat Tardive Dyskinesia but none of them have been completely satisfactory. When it was found that the condition results from a failure in the brain nerve cells to release enough acetylcholine, doctors at Stamford University in America fed choline to a patient with Tardive Dyskinesia to see if it would help. Their experiments were successful and led other researchers, including Dr Wurtman and Dr John Growdon, to carry out more detailed studies. Eventually the results of a carefully controlled study were published in the *New England Journal of Medicine* reporting that nine patients fed choline for two weeks showed major improvements. The ability of choline and lecithin to suppress the distressing movements in Tardive Dyskinesia have since been confirmed in double blind crossover studies and is now widely accepted.

Many other disorders appear to be associated with a lack of acetylcholine in the brain. Preliminary research indicates that lecithin may benefit some patients with Friedreich's Ataxia and Huntington's Chorea. Another disease affecting many elderly people is Alzheimer's Disease, a type of dementia which is characterized by memory disorders, and lecithin is also being tested in patients with Mania since this mood disorder also shows a marked response.

Studies on rats have shown that lecithin and choline can improve short-term memory and the ability to learn. Choline and lecithin are being used to try to see if it is possible to prevent memory loss amongst people suffering from certain kinds of senility.

All this work is very new and scientists do not want to raise false hopes, but it is clear from the findings which have already been reported that our daily food choice can affect the brain. It is likely that the use of lecithin will increase as scientists examine its effect in many other diseases characterized by the failure of the brain to produce enough acetylcholine.

9.
EAT YOUR WAY
TO A HEALTHY HEART

Dietary fats are one of the principal causes of high blood cholesterol and triglyceride levels and, since there is a direct relationship between high blood fat levels and the death rate from coronary heart disease, it makes sound commonsense to attempt, by dietary methods, to reduce these levels. Not only does the average person consume too much fat, many people are also eating too much of the wrong sort of fat. The hard, saturated fats tend to raise blood cholesterol and the liquid or semi-liquid polyunsaturated fats lower the levels. The following section is designed to help the reader plan a lower cholesterol way to a healthy heart by explaining how to reduce total fat consumption and to substitute polyunsaturated fats for dangerous ones. This, however, does not eliminate the need for a daily lecithin supplement, for lecithin has far too important a role to play in the management of fats within the body to be left out. What a low saturated fat diet will do is help lecithin to play its part effectively and, by increasing the amount of essential fatty acids in the diet, ensure that the body itself produces polyunsaturated lecithin.

I hope that this advice will help all who have to follow a low fat diet, whether it be to protect the heart, liver or nerves, or in order to lose weight.

Changing the balance of fats in the diet does not mean a dramatic change in the food eaten since fat is essential – the problem only begins when too much fat of the wrong sort is consumed. It means cutting down on some foods, such as butter, eggs and meat, substituting special margarines, vegetable oils, more fresh fruit and vegetables, and, because it is so important, ensuring that the body receives sufficient of that most vital fat fighting nutrient – pure vegetable lecithin.

General Recommendations

Special reports from scientific bodies all over the world make very similar recommendations for the reduction of total blood cholesterol and other dietary fats in the blood. The Australian Academy of Science, the Royal College of Physicians of London and the Cardiac Society give almost identical advice.

1. A substantial reduction in the total amount of fat in the diet so that it accounts for only about 35 per cent of total calories. At present over 40 per cent of calories come from fat.

2. The type of fat to be limited should be the saturated fats from animal sources, or hardened (hydrogenated) vegetable and marine oils.

3. In order to reduce cholesterol levels it will also be necessary to replace some of the saturated fats with polyunsaturated fats.

4. A general reduction in the total calories from all sources is desirable, especially for those who are over-weight. This will require a reduction in the consumption of carbohydrates as well as fat, since refined carbohydrates, especially sugar and alcohol, are converted into fat if they are not required for energy production.

Most of the fat we eat comes from meat, dairy produce, margarine, cooking fats and cakes and pastries, so a reduction in these would cut down on total fat intake. The Royal College of Physicians report offers further advice in order to reduce saturated fats.

(a) Eat less meat and fewer egg yolks. Eat more poultry and fish. Choose lean meat and remove visible fat from meat. Grill rather than fry.

(b) Use butter sparingly. Preferably use a soft margarine high in polyunsaturated fats. In general avoid cream and the top of the milk.

(c) Use oils rich in polyunsaturated fats for cooking, e.g. corn oil, sunflower oil, safflower oil. Avoid hard margarine or lard. Oils labelled merely 'vegetable oil' may contain a good deal of saturated fat and very little polyunsaturated fat and should be avoided.

(d) Eat more vegetables and fruit.

Copies of the report *Prevention of Coronary Heart Disease* which is reprinted from the Journal of the Royal College of Physicians of London are available from the college in London N.W.1.

The emphasis then is both on a reduction of saturated fats and an increase in polyunsaturates. Since granular soya lecithin is a very rich source of the essential poly-unsaturated fatty acids, linolenic acids, it is an ideal way to implement the recommendations made throughout the world by leading authorities. And remember that because the polyunsaturates in lecithin are in the form of phospho-lipids, they can be used by the body quickly and efficiently.

The following table (reproduced by permission of G.R. Lane Health Products Ltd) lists some popular foods according to their cholesterol levels.

The letters in parenthesis indicate the content of saturated fat. (L) = low, (M) = medium, (H) = high.

Items marked * are free from saturated fats but are easily converted into triglycerides which increase blood fat levels.

High Cholesterol	Medium Cholesterol
Butter (H)	Bacon (lean) (H)
Cakes (H)	Cheese (made with
Crab, lobster, shellfish (L)	wholemilk (H)
Cream (H)	Chicken (L)
Eggs (whole) (L)	Chocolate (M)
Eggs (yolk) (L)	Ice cream (H)
Eggs (fried in butter) (M)	Fish (L)
Omelette (H)	Lard (H)
Fatty meat and bacon (H)	Milk (H)
Kidney (L)	Pancakes (M)
Liver (L)	Poultry (L)
Pastry (H)	Sausages (H)
Soufflés (H)	Veal (M)

Low Cholesterol
Biscuits (M)
Clear soups (L)
Cottage cheese (L)
Margarines (special
    soft) (L)
Skim milk (L)

Coffee and tea
    (no milk) (–)
Fruit (most) (–)
*Honey (–)
*Jam (–)
Nuts (L)
Peanuts (M)
Pasta (L)
*Spirits, wines and
    beer (–)
*Sugar (–)

Cholesterol Free
*Bread and cereals (L)
Coconut (H)

Vegetables (–)
Vegetable oil (L)

The above table can be summarized to give the following guidelines to eating your way to a healthier heart.

Do not use butter or hard margarine for spreading.
Instead, use a soft margarine high in polyunsaturated fats.

Avoid lard, butter or hard margarine in cooking and baking.
Replace them with corn or sunflower oil and poly-unsaturated margarine.

Eat less meat, especially fatty, streaky bacon and organ meats.
Cut the fat from meat and grill rather than fry. Eat more fish and poultry instead of meat. Beware of fat produced in cooking meat (no rich sauces or gravies).

Restrict the use of cream and full cream milk.
Substitute skimmed milk whenever possible for drinking and cooking.

Cut down on eggs and cheese.
Eat no more than three eggs a week and eat cottage or skimmed milk cheeses.

Restrict the number of commercially made cakes and pastries.
Home made cakes and pastries can be made with suitable fats.

Cut down on refined carbohydrates, especially sugar and alcohol.
Eat more fruit and vegetables. Sweeten with honey or molasses.

When dining out try to avoid pâtès, cheese, cream, eggs, rich soups and sauces, fatty meats.

Choose fruit juice, melon or clear soup to start, eat lean cuts of meat, poultry or fish, include fresh vegetables when possible, finish with fruit.

Remember that it is the reduction of total fat intake over a period of time which is important. Do not be too drastic and occasionally make the odd exception if you cannot resist something special – but remember, if you do, the only person you cheat is yourself. Choose the lecithin supplement which is going to be most effective and convenient to take. The granular soya lecithin previously described is the type most often recommended.

Planning and shopping for a low cholesterol/saturated fat diet is not easy without some experience and knowledge of the various types of food eaten. For the housewife and those who regularly eat out at business lunches and social functions, choosing the right food will not be too difficult if the following rules are observed. For convenience these are listed under headings according to the type of food.

Meat, Poultry, Fish
Eat

Lean meat, with all visible fat removed.
Lean beef roasts and steaks.
Roast leg or loin of lamb, lean leg chops.
Veal contains less saturated fat than most meats.
Poultry.
Fresh and salt water fish (not skin).

Avoid

Fatty meat like brisket, spare ribs, mutton, mince, chops.
Pork, as it tends to be fatty.
Processed meats such as sausages, luncheon meat, corned beef, pies, pâté.
Bacon and ham, especially streaky bacon.
Organ meats such as liver and kidney.
Crab, lobster, prawns, all shellfish.

Do not buy ready-cooked canned or frozen meats, there is no way of knowing how much fat they contain.

Always choose lean cuts of meat, avoid cuts which have fat distributed throughout, cut off all visible fats.

When making soups, stews, gravies etc from meat and meat stock, prepare in advance and allow to cool so that the fat hardens and can easily be removed from the surface.

Grill rather than fry. If you must fry, use vegetable oil and avoid basting.

If you must use mince make sure that you see the cut before it is put through the mincer and make sure that it is lean.

Liver is rich in minerals and vitamins and should not be completely eliminated. Serve occasionally but avoid frying.

Meat pies, especially pork pies, contain saturated fats, in both the meat and the pastry.

Remember that fish and poultry are good protein foods and contain less harmful cholesterol and fats than red meats.

Textured vegetable protein can be used as a substitute for meat in many dishes, either as a complete or a partial replacement. Made from soya and with a high protein content, these meat substitutes are available as mince or 'chunks'. They can be helpful in keeping cholesterol and saturated fats out of the food eaten, while still offering variety and texture.

Fats and Oils
Eat
Margarines rich in polyunsaturates. (*Flora, Alfonal Supersoft, St Michael Superspreader* are recommended).
Vegetable oil – corn, safflower, sunflower, soyabean, wheat germ oil are all good provided they have not been hydrogenated.
Salad dressings etc made from the above oils.

Avoid
Butter and hard margarines, lard, suet, meat dripping.
Coconut oil and fat.
Hardened or hydrogenated vegetable oils and shortenings.
Commercially produced cakes and pastries.

Remember that the liquid or semi-solid vegetable oils are

those which contain the polyunsaturates. Avoid vegetable oils and products in which the polyunsaturates have been destroyed by hydrogenation.

Coconut oil, although vegetable, is very saturated.

Always use vegetable oils for frying and browning meat and vegetables.

Use vegetable oil and fat in baking and cooking whenever possible. Do not forget that commercially made cakes and pastries contain a lot of fat. If you bake your own, include oil and special margarines in place of butter.

When frying with vegetable oils use lower temperatures, do not allow the oil to smoke and try to use the oil once only.

Your health food store will stock a variety of suitable oils. Do not be afraid to ask for all the information you need to make sure that the oil you use is rich in polyunsaturates.

Milk, Eggs and Cheese

Eat

Skimmed milk.

Yogurt made with skimmed milk.

Low fat natural yogurt.

Cottage cheese and cheese made with skimmed milk.

Egg whites.

Avoid

Milk and cream.

Egg yolks.

Dairy ice cream.

Chocolate.

Cheese made from whole milk.

Almost all dairy products contain cholesterol and saturated fats. Always use skimmed milk for drinks and in baking.

Avoid cream and evaporated milk. Creamers for coffee often contain coconut fat or hydrogenated oils. They may be free from cholesterol but can be high in saturated fats.

Eat cottage cheeses or cheeses made from skimmed milk. The whole milk cheeses contain both cholesterol and saturated fat.

Limit egg yolks to three per week. They are rich in many vitamins and provide a good source of protein, but they do contain large amounts of cholesterol and they should be strictly limited.

Poaching or boiling eggs avoids the use of fat in their preparation. If you make omelettes or fry, use vegetable oil. Egg whites do not contain harmful fats and can be eaten.

Desserts and Pastry

Eat

Fresh fruit and fruit canned without sugar.
Custard and desserts made with skimmed milk.
Water ices, jellies.
Meringues, home made pies and pastries.

Avoid

Commercially produced pies and cake.
Sweets and desserts containing coconut.
Cream and milk based puddings.
Chocolate puddings and sauces.
Dairy ice cream.

Most fruit is fat-free, although avocado pears do contain some fat and should be eaten in moderation.

Freezing does not adversely affect fruit but most canned fruit contains a high proportion of sugar.

Cream and cream-based desserts contain fat and cholesterol and should be avoided.

Most commercially made biscuits contain saturated fats.

Doughnuts, fritters, pancakes, soufflés should all be avoided.

Vegetables

Fresh vegetables can be eaten with no worries about fat and cholesterol, but resist the temptation to add a pat of butter.

Potatoes are a good wholesome food, but beware of roast potatoes, chips, french fried or potato crisps unless they have been prepared with vegetable oils.

Nuts are a good source of protein and polyunsaturated

oils. Coconut is the exception, as it is highly saturated, and products containing coconut and palm oil (another saturated oil) should be avoided.

Bread and Cereals
Bread and cereal products are usually low in saturated fats. Wholewheat bread and whole grain cereals are preferable because they contain the natural seed germ oils.

Drinks
Fruit juices, tea and coffee are free from fat but avoid adding cream or whole milk. Use skimmed milk instead.

Alcohol is fat free but, because it is a refined carbohydrate, it adds to the body's store of depot fat.

Coffee contains caffeine which can be over-stimulating to the heart and decaffeinated or dandelion coffee is preferable.

Beverages containing cocoa and eggs contain saturated fats. Night time beverages should always be made with skimmed milk.

If drinks have to be sweetened use fructose (fruit sugar) or honey in place of white sugar.

Coffee creamers are free from animal fats but many do contain coconut or palm oil. So check before you use them.

Cooking at Home
The only certain way to know what goes into the food you eat is, of course, to prepare it yourself. Every cook has a favourite recipe and every family their likes and dislikes, but a lot of these dishes will contain eggs, butter, cheese, cream and other saturated fats. This is not a recipe book (there are now some excellent low fat, cholesterol-free cookery books available from health stores, bookshops and most libraries), but here are a few suggestions to encourage you to think and cook the cholesterol-free way.

SOUPS

The basic requirement for most home-made soups is a good stock. Vegetable, chicken or veal are the best as they contain less fat than most other meat stocks. Make the soup the day before it is required and allow it to cool, so that the fat which comes to the surface can be easily removed. If you cannot make it the day before, then cool it quickly in the refrigerator and remove the fat as before.

Cream of Mushroom (or Asparagus) Soup

Imperial (Metric)	American
1 tablespoonful vegetable oil	1 tablespoonful vegetable oil
2 tablespoonsful wholemeal flour	2 tablespoonsful wholewheat flour
1 medium-sized tin of mushrooms or asparagus	1 medium-sized can of mushrooms or asparagus
1 pint (570ml) skimmed milk	2½ cupsful skimmed milk
1 cupful water	1¼ cupsful water
Sea salt and freshly ground black pepper	Sea salt and freshly ground black pepper

1. Heat the vegetable oil and gradually stir in the flour.

2. Add the liquid from the can of vegetables, the milk and water and boil until it thickens, stirring regularly.

3. Add the mushrooms (or asparagus) thinly sliced. Add salt and pepper to taste.

4. Simmer for 10 to 15 minutes. Thin with more water or milk if required.

Vegetable Soup

Imperial (Metric)	American
Piece of knuckle of veal	Piece of knuckle of veal
1 turnip	1 turnip
2 medium-sized carrots	2 medium-sized carrots
1 medium-sized onion	1 medium-sized onion
1 tomato	1 tomato
1 large potato	1 large potato
Celery	Celery
Sea salt and freshly ground black pepper	Sea salt and freshly ground black pepper

1. Place the meat in a large pan or pot three-quarters full of water.

2. Grate the turnips, carrots and onion, slice the peeled tomato, potato and celery and add the vegetables to the pan.

3. Bring to the boil and hold for 2 or 3 minutes whilst removing the scum. Cover and simmer for 2 or 3 hours. Season to taste.

4. When cold remove any surplus fat floating on the surface. Reheat before serving.

Chicken Soup

Imperial (Metric)	American
2½-3 lb (1.25 kilo) chicken	2½-3 pound chicken
1 onion	1 onion
1 bayleaf	1 bayleaf
1 large carrot (grated)	1 large carrot (grated)
Sea salt and freshly ground black pepper	Sea salt and freshly ground black pepper
Parsley	Parsley

1. Clean chicken well and remove as much fat as possible.

2. Place in a large saucepan three-quarters full of water, together with vegetables and bayleaf (include the giblets). Boil until the chicken is tender.

3. Remove chicken and brown in oven. Continue boiling remainder for a further 2 hours.

4. Strain and allow to cool. Remove fat, as in Vegetable Soup, before serving.

FISH

Remember that wet fish is best and that shellfish, crab, lobster, prawns, etc. should be avoided or at least restricted. When fish is fried always use corn or sunflower oil.

Grilled Fish

Take sufficient pieces of fish (sole, halibut, cod, etc.) and season with salt and pepper. Brush on both sides with corn or sunflower oil. Grill until tender. Garnish with parsley before serving.

Fish Cakes

Imperial (Metric)	American
¾lb (340g) potatoes	¾ pound potatoes
1 lb (455g) white fish (boiled)	1 pound white fish (boiled)
Sea salt and freshly ground black pepper	Sea salt and freshly ground black pepper
Milk (hot)	Milk (hot)
Finely chopped parsley, if required	Finely chopped parsley, if required
1 tablespoonful vegetable oil	1 tablespoonful vegetable oil

1. Boil the potatoes in salted water, mash and add the flaked fish. Season to taste, add a little hot milk and oil and mix until creamy.

2. Shape the mixture into flat cakes using a little flour.

3. Fry in hot vegetable oil until brown on both sides.

Haddock Provençale

Imperial (Metric)	American
1 lb (455g) haddock (filleted)	1 pound haddock (filleted)
1 oz (30g) cornflour	¼ cupful cornstarch
Sea salt and freshly ground black pepper	Sea salt and freshly ground black pepper
3 tablespoonsful vegetable oil	3 tablespoonsful vegetable oil
2 large tomatoes	2 large tomatoes
4 oz (115g) sliced mushrooms	1½ cupsful sliced mushrooms
Parsley (chopped for garnish)	Parsley (chopped for garnish)

1. Skin the haddock and cut into small squares. Coat with cornflour and seasoning. Fry in heated oil for 7 to 10 minutes. Remove the fish and keep hot.

2. Skin and slice the tomatoes and add these and the mushrooms to the oil and cook until the mushrooms are done (about 5 minutes).

3. Place the mixture over the fish, garnish with parsley if required, and serve.

MEAT

Probably the most important part of the preparation of meat dishes is the selection of the piece of meat to be used. Make sure that it contains as little fat as possible and remove all visible fat before starting to cook. Avoid choosing cuts with fat running through them as this is almost impossible to remove. Veal is probably the leanest meat and is recommended. It is difficult to remove the fat from mutton so it is best avoided. Chicken is low in fat but the skin should be discarded. When roasting meat season the joint of meat to be used and put a little vegetable oil in the roasting pan. Do not use lard or animal fats.

Beef and Mushroom Casserole

Imperial (Metric)	*American*
1 lb (455 g) stewing steak	1 pound stewing steak
1 oz (30 g) cornflour	¼ cupful cornstarch
Sea salt and freshly ground black pepper	Sea salt and freshly ground black pepper
2 onions (sliced)	2 onions (sliced)
2 tablespoonsful vegetable oil	2 tablespoonsful vegetable oil
2 carrots (sliced)	2 carrots (sliced)
2 beef stock cubes	2 beef stock cubes
1 pint (570 ml) water	2½ cupsful water
2 peppers (red or green)	2 peppers (red or green)
2 oz (55 g) mushrooms (sliced)	2 oz (55 g) mushrooms (sliced)

1. Remove fat from heat and cut into cubes. Coat with cornflour and season with salt and pepper.

2. Gently fry the meat and onions in the oil at the bottom of the dish, add the carrots and beef stock. Bring to the boil, stirring well.

3. Cover and simmer for 1 hour or until the meat is tender. After about 45 minutes add the peppers and mushrooms.

Goulash

Imperial (Metric)	*American*
1 lb (455 g) stewing steak	1 pound stewing steak
1 onion	1 onion
¾ lb (350 g) tomatoes	12 ounces tomatoes
1 oz (30 g) polyunsaturated margarine	2½ tablespoonsful polyunsaturated margarine
Flour seasoned with black pepper, salt and paprika	Flour seasoned with black pepper, salt and paprika
½ pint (285 ml) beef stock	1⅓ cupsful beef stock
Pinch mixed herbs	Pinch mixed herbs
Small carton of low fat natural yogurt	Small carton of low fat natural yogurt

1. Remove fat from meat and cut into small pieces.

2. Peel and chop the onions and slice the tomatoes. Fry the onions in margarine until they are clear.

3. Season the meat with flour and add to the onions, fry for about 10 minutes until brown. Add remaining ingredients except yogurt and bring to the boil.

4. Place in casserole, cover and cook for 2 to 2½ hours in the centre of the oven at 325°F/170°C (Gas Mark 3).

5. Just before serving stir in the yogurt. Garnish with parsley if required.

LIGHT MEALS

Cholesterol Free Pastry

Imperial (Metric)	*American*
8 oz (225 g) plain wholemeal flour	2 cupsful plain wholewheat flour
Pinch of sea salt	Pinch of sea salt
4 oz (100 g) polyunsaturated margarine	½ cupful polyunsaturated margarine
2 tablespoonsful cold water	2 tablespoonsful cold water

1. Sieve the flour and salt into a mixing bowl.

2. Rub the margarine into the flour until it forms a crumb-like mixture.

3. Mix in the water to form a firm dough. Knead gently on a floured board. Roll out and use as required.

This will produce enough pastry to line a 7 in (18cm)-8 in (20cm) flan dish.

Cheese and Salmon Quiche

Imperial (Metric)	American
Cholesterol free pastry	Cholesterol free pastry
1 egg	1 egg
¼ pint (140ml) milk	⅔ cupful milk
Sea salt and freshly ground black pepper	Sea salt and freshly ground black pepper
Small onion	Small onion
3oz (85g) cheese (grated)	¾ cupful cheese (grated)
7oz (200g) tin salmon or tuna fish	Small can salmon or tuna fish

1. Roll out pastry thinly and line 4 individual 4 in (10cm) flan rings or an 8 in (20cm) flan ring.

2. Whisk the egg and milk with a little salt and pepper.

3. Peel and grate the onion and mix the onions and cheese with the egg and milk.

4. Drain the fish and flake, divide it between the pastry cases. Spoon the cheese mixture over the top.

5. Bake for 15 minutes at 400°F/200°C (Gas Mark 6). Reduce to 350°F/180°C (Gas Mark 4) for a further 25 minutes until golden brown. Garnish with parsley and serve hot or cold.

Mushroom à la Grecque

Imperial (Metric)	American
1 onion	1 onion
2 tablespoonsful vegetable oil	2 tablespoonsful vegetable oil
1 clove garlic	1 clove garlic
¼ pint (140 ml) dry white wine	⅔ cupful dry white wine
Sea salt and freshly ground black pepper	Sea salt and freshly ground black pepper
1 lb (455 g) button mushrooms	8 cupsful button mushrooms
½ lb (225 g) tomatoes	8 ounces tomatoes
Bouquet garni	Bouquet garni
Chopped parsley	Chopped parsley

1. Peel and finely chop the onions and cook over a low heat in the oil until soft but not coloured.

2. Peel but do not chop the garlic. Add the wine, garlic and other ingredients to the onions.

SWEETS

Fresh fruit is often the best choice to end a meal. This is especially true of eating out, when many of those attractive sweets are full of saturated fats and cholesterol. With a little imagination delicious low cholesterol, low fat sweets can be served.

Lemon Pudding

Imperial (Metric)	American
2 tablespoonsful vegetable oil	2 tablespoonsful vegetable oil
4 oz (100 g) raw cane sugar	⅔ cupful raw cane sugar
1 lemon	1 lemon
1 tablespoonful wholemeal flour	1 tablespoonful wholewheat flour
1 cupful skimmed milk	1¼ cupsful skimmed milk
2 egg whites	2 egg whites

1. Mix oil and sugar well. Add a little grated lemon rind and the juice of the lemon and mix well.

2. Add flour and stir. Mix in the milk. Stiffly beat the egg whites and stir into the mixture. Pour onto an oiled dish.

3. Place in a pan of water and bake at 350°F/180°C (Gas Mark 4) for 45 minutes or until golden brown.

Marmalade Tart

Imperial (Metric)	*American*
¾lb (340g) cholesterol-free pastry (page 86)	12 ounces cholesterol-free pastry (page 86)
2oz (55g) polyunsaturated margarine	¼ cupful polyunsaturated margarine
1oz (30g) fine ground raw cane sugar	2 tablespoonsful fine ground raw cane sugar
1 egg	1 egg
1 tablespoonful wholemeal flour	1 tablespoonful wholewheat flour
2 tablespoonsful thick-cut marmalade	2 tablespoonsful thick-cut marmalade

1. Line an 8in (20cm) flan dish with pastry. Prick the bottom of the pastry case and cover with greaseproof paper and fill with dry crusts or beans. Bake for 15 minutes at 400°F/200°C (Gas Mark 6).

2. Mix the margarine and sugar until light and fluffy. Beat in the egg. Use a tablespoon to fold in the flour and the marmalade.

3. Remove the pastry from the oven and remove the filling and greaseproof paper.

4. Spoon in filling. Lower the oven to 360°F/180°C (Gas Mark 4). Cook for 30 minutes. Allow to cool slightly before removing tart from dish onto a warm serving plate. Serve hot.

Pancakes

Imperial (Metric)	*American*
1 egg white	1 egg white
1 cupful wholemeal flour	1¼ cupsful wholewheat flour
Sea salt and freshly ground black pepper	Sea salt and freshly ground black pepper
2 tablespoonsful water	2 tablespoonsful water
¾ cupful skimmed milk	1 cupful skimmed milk
½ teaspoonful baking powder	½ teaspoonful baking soda
1 tablespoonful raw cane sugar	1 tablespoonful raw cane sugar

1. Mix egg white and flour together with a pinch of salt. Add water and milk and mix until smooth and free from lumps. Add the baking powder.

2. Put enough oil to just cover the base of a frying pan. Pour in a thin layer of mix and fry lightly on both sides.

3. Remove from pan, spread honey or other filling on one side then fold over.

Be bold and experiment, you will find that it is possible to make delicious meals and still avoid the dangers of the high fat, high cholesterol foods.

GLOSSARY OF TERMS USED

Angina pectoris. A severe, sudden, vice-like pain in the chest over the heart caused by a reduction in the blood supply. Often occurs when the coronary arteries, which supply blood to the heart, are narrowed by atherosclerosis and the heart muscle has to overcome resistance.

Anti-oxidant. Fat, especially polyunsaturated fat, is subject to spoilage, known as rancidity, when oxygen is present. This process can be retarded by the presence of 'anti-oxidants' which preserve the food. Vitamin E, vitamin C and garlic are natural anti-oxidants for fats.

Arteriosclerosis. The thickening and narrowing of the artery walls caused by deposits of cholesterol and other fats often known as 'hardening of the arteries'. It is a term used to describe a variety of conditions that cause the artery walls to become thick and lose their elasticity.

Atherosclerosis. A type of arteriosclerosis which occurs in the inner walls of the arteries carrying blood to the heart (the coronary arteries). Fatty deposits, such as cholesterol, build up on the inside of the artery, reducing the supply of blood to the heart. It is a major cause of fatal heart disease.

Cholesterol. A fat-like substance present throughout the body and in all animal tissues. It is needed by the body for many purposes and becomes dangerous to health when present in excess in the blood. High blood cholesterol levels are associated with heart disease. Cholesterol is deposited on the artery wall and causes atherosclerosis (see above). Gallstones consist of over 90 per cent cholesterol.

Choline. A vitamin belonging to the vitamin B group. It is believed to be very important to the liver in the metabolism of fat. It is present in lecithin in the form of phosphatidyl choline, the phospholipid found in great concentration in the heart.

Coronary thrombosis. A thrombosis is a clot which forms in the blood, caused by platelets sticking together. When it occurs in the coronary arteries it is known as coronary thrombosis and can be fatal.

Depot fat. Fat which is not immediately used by the body is stored in the tissues as depot fat until it is required to produce energy. Excess refined carbohydrates, such as alcohol and sugar, are converted into depot fat.

Essential fatty acids and fatty acids. Fatty acids are used to build fats such as the triglycerides. They may be saturated or unsaturated (see opposite). The most saturated are linoleic, linolenic and arachidonic acids. These are called essential fatty acids because they are needed for good health, but cannot be made within the body and so, like vitamins, must be present in the diet. The essential fatty acids occur mostly in polyunsaturated vegetable oils.

Hydrogenation. A process used to change a liquid poly-unsaturated oil into a more solid saturated one. It is used to prevent rancidity and to harden vegetable oils in the production of some margarines and shortenings. It has the effect of reducing the essential fatty acid content of vegetable oils. Oils can be lightly hydrogenated so that they remain liquid, and these are sometimes described as being 'specially processed'.

Inositol. Like choline, a B group vitamin. The whole of the B complex is important in the metabolism of fats, and inositol (together with choline) is especially concerned with fat and cholesterol.

Lecithin. Is a complex mixture of phospholipids consisting of essential fatty acids, choline, inositol and phosphorus. It is present in both animal and vegetable cells and is capable of emulsifying fats and water. The most important function of lecithin concerns the control of cholesterol and other fats in the body. Vegetable lecithin, usually obtained from soya beans, is an important source of essential polyunsaturated fatty acids. The most highly recommended type as a nutritional supplement is in a granular form of very pure lecithin.

Lipids. The scientific name given to dietary oils and fats. They occur in foods in two forms. First, the depot or storage lipids which are reserve energy supplies forming the bulk of fat in the body. The second form is the more complex lipids used in the structure of cells. They play a key role in the regulation of many processes which take place in the body.

Metabolism. The chemical routine of the body. A host of complicated chemical processes are constantly taking place within the human body, converting the food we eat and drink and the air we breathe into the form needed to maintain health, provide energy and build new body cells. These processes are known as the metabolism.

Mono-unsaturated fats. Fatty acids are distinguished by the number of carbon atoms and 'double bonds' which the contain. Those with one double bond are mono-unsaturated, the most common being oleic acid. They have little or no effect on raising or lowering blood cholesterol levels.

Polyunsaturated fats. Because they have more double bonds available than the other fatty acids, some fats can absorb additional hydrogen, making them capable of reacting and linking with other nutrients in the body. The poly-unsaturates have two or more double bonds available and, because they are not normally produced by the body itself, they are known as essential fatty acids. The poly-unsaturated fats tend to lower blood cholesterol levels and are recommended as a partial substitute for saturated fats to reduce accumulations of fatty deposits in the arteries. They are usually liquid vegetable oils. Lecithin is a rich source of polyunsaturates.

Saturated fats. Some fats cannot absorb any additional hydrogen and are said to be saturated. They are usually of animal origin, such as meat, butter, egg yolk. Hardened or hydrogenated vegetable oils become saturated. These fats should be restricted because they increase the amount of cholesterol in the blood.

Triglycerides. Most food fats consist largely of the tri-glycerides which contain three fatty acids linked with a unit of glycerine. It is the principal form in which fat exists in the body and is used mainly for energy storage. Like cholesterol, triglycerides are believed to be responsible for arterial and heart disease.

INDEX